Elaine Leong Eng, MD

A Christian Approach to Overcoming Disability
A Doctor's Story

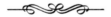
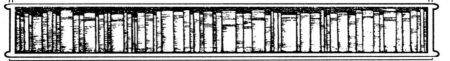

More pre-publication
REVIEWS, COMMENTARIES, EVALUATIONS . . .

"This is a touching and very encouraging book written by a Christian psychiatrist and obstetrician/gynecologist who has been able to live a full life despite her blindness that happened seven years into her marriage. Her faith in God and His Word shine through her stories. Dr. Elaine Eng has written a book that will deeply bless and enrich all of us, whether we have disabilities or not. I highly recommend it!"

Reverend Siang-Yang Tan, PhD
Professor of Psychology,
Fuller Theological Seminary;
Senior Pastor, First Evangelic Church,
Glendale, California

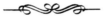

"You will laugh, cry, and be nourished by Dr. Elaine Eng's spiritual medicine in her new book. It is what you get when you cross Edith Schaeffer with Amy Tan—quirky, wise, and humane. Her obsessions are as funny as they are inspiring. Her telling of "The Mop Story" and "The Cane Memory" will give you so much funny love that you will want to cry.

Decked out in an orange and black tank top, pink sweatpants, red Reebok high-top sneakers, and a 'real white cane,' Dr. Eng guides us through life's rejections, panics, anxieties, irrational fears, and exhaustions with zestful encouragements. She shows the funny spiritual side of accidentally putting green scrubby sponges in her husband's soup, acetone cotton balls in his Coke, kitty litter on his bath towel, and pink dye on his underwear.

Just when all your sensibilities are jangled to aliveness, this blind psychiatrist hits you with sumptuous recipes of goulash, soup, apple pie, and Navajo fry bread. After you finish this book, you will feel like you have just had a savory meal and are ready to conquer the world with fun, love, laughter, and a deeper soul."

Dr. Tony Carnes
Senior News Writer, *Christianity Today;*
Chair, Seminar on Contents
and Methods in the Social Sciences,
Columbia University; Director,
Research Institute for New Americans

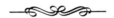

"Readers will be particularly interested in how this highly professional woman, an obstetrician/gynecologist and psychiatrist, understands the true meaning of being 'submissive' to her husband and putting her family first, while she manages a private counseling practice, is active in her church and local pregnancy resource center, teaches in a master's program, and travels to foreign missions—all with the help of her 'seeing-eye' white cane! And all with a humility and grace that is truly inspiring!

Readers, although perhaps not technically 'disabled,' will relate to Dr. Eng's doubts about whether her husband sees her as 'damaged goods' and whether her teenagers are embarrassed when they are seen with her. She weaves into her personal stories of doubts, fears, and triumphs the inspiring threads of scripture, giving deeper meaning (literal and figurative) to the many verses on 'sight' and 'blindness.' This is a fascinating personal story of the rewards of living by faith and not by sight."

Margaret H. Hartshorn, PhD
President, Heartbeat International

More pre-publication
REVIEWS, COMMENTARIES, EVALUATIONS . . .

"This is an engaging account of triumph through tragedy, a personal exemplification of Paul's words: 'Our light affliction, which is but for a moment, works for us a far more exceeding and eternal weight of glory' (2 Corinthians 4:17)."

Norman L. Geisler, PhD
President,
Southern Evangelical Seminary,
North Carolina

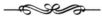

"Dr. Elaine Eng's book provides an insightful look into the moral and spiritual fiber of one who turned a physical challenge into a blessing, not only for herself but for countless others. Having sight and then losing it provides the author opportunities to share her deep faith and courage with others who endure physical, mental, or emotional challenges of their own.

Dr. Eng teaches us that, like the willow tree, we must bend with the winds in order to remain confident and firmly planted in the place where we should be. Her seven steps for dealing with anxiety and worries should be clipped and placed on the refrigerator for a constant reminder that, although worries and anxiety do come, they can be dealt with effectively. How? By focusing our attention to the sovereign God who provides comfort and aid—in everything."

Gerald D. Swim
Academic Officer, Christian Medical
& Dental Association's
International Continuing Medical
& Dental Education Conferences

The Haworth Pastoral Press®
An Imprint of The Haworth Press
New York • London • Oxford

A Christian Approach to Overcoming Disability
A Doctor's Story

THE HAWORTH PASTORAL PRESS
Religion and Mental Health
Harold G. Koenig, MD
Senior Editor

A Christian Approach to Overcoming Disability
A Doctor's Story

Elaine Leong Eng, MD

The Haworth Pastoral Press®
An Imprint of The Haworth Press, Inc.
New York • London • Oxford

Published by

The Haworth Pastoral Press®, an imprint of The Haworth Press, Inc., 10 Alice Street, Binghamton, NY 13904-1580.

Scripture taken from the HOLY BIBLE, NEW INTERNATIONAL VERSION. NIV. Copyright © 1973, 1978, 1984 by International Bible Society. Used by permission of Zondervan. All rights reserved.

Scripture taken from the NEW AMERICAN STANDARD BIBLE®, Copyright © 1960, 1962, 1963, 1968, 1971, 1972, 1973, 1975, 1977, 1995 by The Lockman Foundation. Used by permission.

Cover design by Lora Wiggins

Library of Congress Cataloging-in-Publication Data

Eng, Elaine Leong.
    A Christian approach to overcoming disability : a doctor's story / Elaine Leong Eng.
        p. cm.
    Includes bibliographical references and index.
    ISBN 0-7890-2257-5 (alk. paper)—ISBN 0-7890-2258-3 (pbk. : alk. paper)
    1. People with disabilities—Religious life. I. Title.
BV4910.E54 2003
248.8'64—dc21
                                                                                    2003012284

This book is dedicated to my parents
Mr. and Mrs. Gwock Jing Leong,
my grandfather Leong,
and my future grandchildren.

ABOUT THE AUTHOR

Elaine Leong Eng, MD, is a physician who changed career specialties from obstetrics and gynecology to psychiatry due to the onset of blindness. Practicing in a field that is attuned to human coping and adaptation, she has identified important issues and beliefs about blindness as it impacts on her profession, family, and identity.

Dr. Eng is a graduate of Princeton University and the Albert Einstein College of Medicine. She is currently Clinical Assistant Professor of Psychiatry in the Department of Obstetrics and Gynecology at Cornell-Weill Medical College and a faculty member at the Alliance Theological Seminary's Graduate School of Counseling. Trained in the Lay Ministry Program of Concordia College, Dr. Eng integrates faith and psychology to provide mental health education. Avenues for this endeavor have included speaking engagements, nationally and internationally. Her first book, *"Martha, Martha": How Christians Worry* (Haworth), is a text on anxiety written for the Christian audience. Dr. Eng serves as President of the Board of Directors at the Boro Pregnancy Counseling Center and is a Distinguished Fellow of the American Psychiatric Association. She is the recipient of the Queens County Psychiatric Society Award and the "Servant Leadership Award" from Heartbeat International.

CONTENTS

Foreword

His disciples asked Him, "Rabbi, who sinned, this man or his parents, that he would be born blind?" Jesus answered, "It was neither that this man sinned, nor his parents, but it was so that the works of God might be displayed in him."

John 9:2,3
New American Standard Bible

Consider it all joy, my brethren, when you encounter various trials.

James 1:2
New American Standard Bible

My first encounter with Elaine Eng came several years ago at an annual meeting of mental health professionals, where I had just given a talk describing opportunities for psychiatrists in foreign mission service. This attractive and animated woman approached, introduced herself, and indicated she was planning to go on a mission trip herself. I was initially disconcerted as she looked past me while speaking; it was several minutes before I realized she was blind. I experienced the expected flood of internal questions and emotions: "Why would such a thing happen to such a lovely person? What is she thinking? How could she possibly even get to the mission field, much less be of value there?" Soon thereafter, I read her first book, *"Martha, Martha": How Christians Worry* (The Haworth Press, 2000), and began a process of understanding that this very special woman, this gifted doctor of both obstetrical and psychiatric expertise, was not someone to be limited or defined by her "impairment."

In *A Christian Approach to Overcoming Disability,* Elaine's journey from sight to sightlessness is recounted from many perspectives. The book examines blindness from her personal experiences as influenced by culture, marriage, family, and the author's role as professor, physician, and mentor. Her travels abroad are described, as are events of the past several years that have brought an awareness of tragedy to all of us. But this book is not about tragedy. It is about triumph.

In my own medical practice, I have known many people who have been faced with what seemed to be overwhelming disabilities or handicaps, and I have been encouraged by their adaptation to their situations. Yet "adaptation" is not a sufficient word for what Elaine has accomplished. Hers is a story of victory—not just victory in spite of her blindness, but victory because of her blindness. This is evidence of the presence and the power of God in her life, as Elaine shows us how to celebrate such a trial, to be grateful for the new opportunities it provides.

This book could have been about a remarkable woman's unusual ability to live life richly in circumstances of potential restriction. Elaine has, in her typical style, given us much more. She has given us a glimpse into the wholeness and abundance of God's grace. In doing so, she has given us hope—hope to approach those restrictions, those limitations, those trials that we ourselves may face in our own lives and find foreboding.

So, fear not. Go ahead, turn the page, gear up, and take the first step. Climb the wall. Go for the goal. And consider it all joy!

Barney M. Davis Jr., MD, FAPA
Executive Director, Godspeed Missionary Care
Chairman, Psychiatry Section, Christian Medical Association

Preface

At Christmastime one year, a visiting youth pastor spoke at our church about the need for encouragement and counseling for young people suffering from despair and hopelessness. A point of interest was the fact that, prior to entering the ministry, he was a psychiatric social worker in a mental health facility. As part of a multidisciplinary team, he treated the psychological, sociological, and other special needs of a metropolitan community largely composed of Chinese immigrants to the United States. Now, as a minister, he has had the opportunity to address similar needs, clearly integrating his mental health training with a theological and spiritual perspective. This was evident to me as he preached his sermon on the topic of "encouragement" to the burdened and afflicted. At the time I did not know of his psychiatric background, but as the sermon unfolded, I detected a clear sense of his adaptation of psychological tools enhanced by a biblical foundation.

Using the acronym LIFE, he outlined four essentials of encouragement. As any well-trained counselor would surmise, the L stands for *Listen*. Listening, and possessing the skills to do it well, is the hallmark of helping those who have unmet emotional needs. Second, he spoke of *Inspiration*. One must somehow be inspirational in a manner that motivates others toward progress and healing. F stands for *Foresee*—help the other person foresee the potential for a better situation, self-image, or outcome. Foreseeing is simply giving the person the vital commodity of hope. Generated by a vision of improving circumstances, a better future achieved by personal and God-given resources, or a sense of significance in the world, hope will offset the empty blackness of despair. Finally, the E stands for *Engage*. The counselor must find some way to engage the person either in a relationship or dialogue that will prompt the afflicted person to make progress. Together the acronym of these action items spells out the word *life*. Jesus said, "I am come that they might have life, and that they might have it more abundantly."[1] It is my hope that the collection of autobiographical essays in this book will offer encouragement through the LIFE tools taught by this youth pastor. Although unable to actually listen to the needs of every reader, I have pointed him or her to an omnipresent God that will. I pray that this book will inspire its audience through the stories that are told. Then, despite my blindness or perhaps because of it, I would like the book to *foresee* a vision of peace, hope, and mastery for those who need it. Finally, I ask the reader to *engage* with me in this book, along with friends and caregivers, to make progress in life's journeys. The minister spoke of the Chinese word for vitamin. It is *way-ta-ming.* When spoken, it sounds similar to the English word, and most believe that this is the derivation of the translation of vitamin. However, if one looks at each Chinese word separately, the individual meanings, when combined, state, "giving others life." There is no better definition for encouragement. May this book be God's *way-ta-ming,* energizing many toward the mastery of trials and challenges.

Acknowledgments

I wish to acknowledge the venerable list of physicians who have inspired, educated, and cared for me: Dr. Ronald Carr, Dr. Phyllis Chang, Dr. Joseph Chiu, Dr. T. Y. Dang, Dr. Margaret Hom Eng, Dr. Maria Finley, Dr. Simon Grolnick, Dr. Lorraine Milio, Dr. Robert Porges, Dr. Robert Post, Dr. Jean Schultz, Dr. Jerry Seiler, Dr. Thornton Vandersall, and Dr. Livia Wan.

Many thanks to Soraya Cina, Nancy Moy, and Nancy Chu for their help in the preparation of the book, and to Alice Ling and the many who have assisted me in my travels.

I am also grateful for the kindness and support of Leonard Holland, Esquire, Lonnie Typond, Reverend Lee Hearn, Reverend Kuo-liang Lin, Rose Chin, Maymay Quey Lin, Elizabeth Dahlberg, Kathleen Brennan, Gerald Brezenoff, and all my friends, students, and church and family members who have helped me meet the challenge.

And above all, I credit my "agent," the Great Physician, the Wonderful Counselor—the Mighty God.

Chapter 1

God Is My Agent

A well-known author advised me to acquire a good agent when I was writing the draft of my first book, *"Martha, Martha": How Christians Worry*. His sincere admonition was based on his own personal experiences of regret at not having done so. Finding such a person was more difficult than I expected, and between trying to juggle writing, raising a family, and maintaining a career in psychiatry, I had to abandon my search for an agent. Nonetheless, I was concerned that my "success" as an author might have been jeopardized by my lack of an advocate in the competitive marketplace of publishing. I was wrong. The following are anecdotes of how God, in His divine providence and often with good humor, became the best agent one can "hire."

On May 15, 2000, I was to receive the honor of being a newly elected fellow to the American Psychiatric Association. This was to be celebrated in a convocation whereby I would be expected to march in a procession with the many other newly elected fellows and place a gold medallion on a cord around my neck in front of a large audience of highly esteemed professionals and dignitaries. Being blind from retinitis pigmentosa, I obsessed over the physical challenges of such a ceremony. The last thing I wanted to do was to call attention to myself more than necessary. I was afraid that I would embarrass myself by stumbling out of line or marching toward the wrong destination. The kind staff person handling this event gave me the option of being seated from the beginning, and I thankfully seized the opportunity. She promptly brought me to a seat where I breathed a sigh of relief. A woman in front of me turned around and introduced herself as the wife of one of the presidential award winners and told me that I was seated in the second row of the auditorium. She was genuinely friendly, and she asked me many questions about myself. Before long, we were having a great conversation. Having learned about my book, she wanted to purchase a copy for her daughter's new father-in-law-to-be, as he was the general secretary of the American Baptist Churches USA. It occurred to me that this serendipitous event was actually God being my "agent," because never in a million years would I have found this warm, receptive woman who was connected to the right resource for promoting my book.

The rest of the program I spent in embarrassment, as I soon realized that I was placed in the wrong seat and had to stand virtually alone, apart from my colleagues, to be recognized as a fellow. I also had to remain seated while the row of distinguished fellows I was misplaced with stood when it was their turn to be honored. You can imagine the confusion experienced by my neighbors when I stubbornly refused to stand when the group I was seated with was asked to rise. Then, the scene became all the more laughable when my own group was asked to stand—and I stood alone in front of Chicago's large convention center, McCormick Place. I must have stuck out like a sore thumb as my colleagues arose about twenty rows behind me. The concluding moment was equally awkward. I was escorted alone in the recessional by a well-meaning but anxious staff person who "jumped the gun" and hurried me down the aisle, *alone,* for all to see. Because he was unaccustomed to assisting visually challenged persons, the way he grabbed me must have looked more like a police officer nabbing a criminal suspect. The scene must have been at least befuddling if not hilarious to a crowd of psychiatrists. This sort of attention was the one thing I had dreaded the most. In retrospect, the snafus of this night's events were more than balanced by the opportunity to share my writing with the leader of a national Christian organization. The following year I received this e-mail, which had been written by him and sent to this same woman I had met at McCormick Place.

Subject: Elaine Leong Eng, MD, Book
Date: 06/20/2001 7:38:15 AM Pacific Daylight Time
From: The Reverend Doctor D. Weiss
To: Donna

Dear Donna,

I have read *Martha Martha* by Elaine Leong Eng . . .
The book seeks to enable Christian churchgoers to be open to the insights and contributions of psychiatry and to enable them to be helpful and supportive, as laypeople, to friends and relatives facing worry, phobias, anxieties, depression, etc.
I think she has produced a volume which can be very helpful to the audience she has in mind. She is balanced in her outlook, writes clearly, and is on the wavelength of her potential readers (i.e., relatively conservative Christian churchgoers).
I think it is a very fine book for what it intends to be. If used it can be a fine tool in helping people.[1]

CONSIDER THE LILIES

Meeting Ausma Mursch (née Ozols), the director of the Lutheran Counseling Center, is like being caught in a dramatic whirlwind, but somehow you have the conviction that, when the weather pattern is over, you will land not only on your feet but also in a better place. A friend had advised me to call the center, where I first had the chance to meet Ausma. She demonstrated an immediate liking to me and a desire to collaborate in mental health education. She planned multiple conferences, affording me excellent opportunities to discuss anxiety, the subject of my book. She also put me in touch with Rich Bimbler, an author and the president of Wheat Ridge Ministries, a national Lutheran organization advocating health and wellness. Finally, she announced that one of the Lutheran pastors supporting the counseling center, Reverend Vernon Schultheis, was about to publish a wonderful review of my book for their newsletter. God surely was doing some "agenting" here. Let me tell you more about Ausma.

Ausma Ozols was born in Riga, Latvia, to a well-respected family that raised their two daughters with strong family values and a deep Christian faith. However, early in the family's life, the political climate in their country changed. At age four, Ausma's father, who was a congressman, had to send her, her sister, and her mother into hiding and eventually to escape to Germany when the Russians invaded their country. He later joined them and decided to have his family work on a German farm in return for housing and food. However, they were eventually put in a German displaced persons refugee camp until they received permission to travel to a final homeland. The camps were dehumanizing, unsanitary, and cramped. Moreover, Germany was being bombed daily, as they were in the middle of World War II. Ausma remembers playing in the rubble of destroyed buildings that had been hit by bombs. She recalls jumping and hiding under anything she could when she heard loud explosions and tells the story of landing in a thistle bush in one of her escape attempts. Her mother later had to remove scores of painful thistle needles from her body. After her transport to the United States under the sponsorship of a Methodist church, Ausma's family industriously adapted to life in Kalamazoo, Michigan, making major contributions to their church and community. Instead of breeding hate and bitterness, Ausma's experiences left her with a strong sense of empathy and compassion for those who are different and in need. She attributes this outcome to her father's steadfast influence in not letting the war experiences destroy their family.

So what does a Latvian war survivor have in common with a Chinese blind psychiatrist? I have personally received the benefits of Ausma's family heritage. Ausma volunteered to sponsor me for a parish nurse conference at Concordia University in Wisconsin. She told many that she was "going to be my eyes on this trip" so that I could be the keynote speaker. She would also do a workshop for the nurses about stress and burnout. In many ways, she acted as my guardian angel, protecting me from dangerous falls and making sure that I got from place to place safely. Angels are one of her favorite things, and she collects representations of them in various art forms. I can see how she patterns herself after them. She has always felt the presence of the cherubim, especially in times of threat or anxiety, as have I. Unlike typical celestial beings, sometimes Ausma acted more as an agent than an angel. I found her promoting my books, my work, and just about anything else she thought I could do for others. When I asked her how she could so easily motivate me to do something when it is not an easy thing to do, she simply said, "It's because I wanted you to do it."

"Yes," I replied, "but many people want me to do things, and I have the good sense and discernment and courage to say no. How do you find a way to hone in and ultimately devise a plan that really works?" In the end, I could not help but say "yes" and really know that it was a good idea.

"It's because I always have a second plan, if the first doesn't work. I feel that I must find a way!"[2] This is quintessential Ausma.

Ausma's attitude toward me is clearly respectful, honoring, and not patronizing, as I have sometimes encountered, being handicapped. The content of her words coming from any other source might be viewed as patronizing, but from her it is not so. She tells me that "Being your eyes is a privilege." She says she spent time with me because she was curious about my faith and how it operated in my life. She wondered if I was genuinely handling my professional life as well as it seemed and how my professed faith contributed to it. I believe that God helped me to demonstrate that to her in Wisconsin—but not through words, as sometimes words fail to truly capture the operation of divine grace in a person's life. Rather, its impact on a person's thoughts and behavior needs to be observed, especially when it is so different from the humanly expected course. Why am I not bitter in my blindness, but rather at ease and even triumphant in its wake? Probably for the same providential reason that Ausma did such loving, caring, extensive work in the aftermath of September 11, 2001. She saw the buildings burn, and she was filled with compassion for the intense pain that would arise from this incident. Never one to avoid a challenge, the fight-or-flight response energized her to work tirelessly after the attack, winning commendations from Governor George Pataki and many others in her faith community for her contributions through the Lutheran Counseling Center. As a child, she remembers playing in the rubble of bombed-out Dresden, Germany; as an adult, she found herself working in the emotional rubble of New York City following 9/11. Only the divine creator can establish such powerful compassion in a person who could have been em-

bittered by the profound losses experienced in war. Yet she concludes that in her life "God's presence is a powerful tool and reason for survival" which has allowed her to pass on love rather than
hate. Her philosophy in life is, "I will find a way," which is analogous to my own belief: "I will work hard to find a way and rely on
the fact that God will make a way." God has done so for this Latvian and Chinese team, so different in background and yet so similar. According to Latvian culture, Ausma was born in the month of
the calla lily, a symbol of hope and life. My own Chinese name
means "brilliant jade." Together, God has used lily and jade to create a still-life portrait of strength, purpose, and dignity. God is
such a masterful artist!

FOOD FOR THOUGHT

One night, an obstetrician who was a medical school classmate
of mine invited me to his home to speak to his Bible study group.
He asked me to share my testimony and discuss my book. A large
crowd of Chinese Christians and their Caucasian friends gathered
at his Long Island home. As with most Asian gatherings, much of
the activity is devoted to the food, and the potluck dishes that night
were spectacular: Shrimp, sautéed flank steak with a potpourri of
vegetables, deliciously seasoned fish, fragrantly spiced meat stews,
and other delicacies covered the large dining table. This was
matched by an equally large and enticing dessert spread that combined the best from both the East and the West. After a meal of
sheer exquisite satiation, we settled down to the program. My audience was ostensibly interested in how to manage anxiety from a
biblical and clinical standpoint, but they were also very interested
in my own personal journey with blindness and how I have coped.
I shared how God helped me accept my diagnosis and how His
grace made it possible for me to transition into my new role with
unusual ease. Some felt that I did not offer enough information
about myself, but there was so much to cover. It is often hard to
speak to a group of strangers and determine what their needs are
and how to address them. Some want information; some want answers to their own individual struggles; some hope that you can

give them the ABCs that will get rid of all anxiety (which is unrealistic); and some are just plain curious. Not having the visual cues of the audience response also makes it more challenging. I am getting better at discerning the needs of groups as I speak. I find that a lengthy question-and-answer period is the best way to learn the agenda of a new audience, and I welcome that part of the talk. By God's grace, the program went so well that I was signing books until midnight!

THE BIRTH OF A BOOK

The most memorable night of my career occurred on February 29, 2000. This night was my "leap" into authorship, as it was the day my book was released and I had the chance to celebrate at the Marriott Marquis Hotel in the exciting Broadway theater district of New York City. The glittering lights of the neon signs streaming through the many restaurant windows and the busy traffic outside provided a wonderful backdrop for the exhilaration I was feeling. It is akin to having just given birth but being physically well and energetic enough to celebrate with gusto. Present at the dinner in the private atmosphere of this midtown restaurant were Mr. William Palmer, director of publications and vice president of The Haworth Press; Dr. Thornton Vandersall, professor emeritus at Cornell University Medical College; Mrs. Debbie Wessely, executive director of the Queens County branch of the American Psychiatric Association; Reverend Curtis Hart, director of Pastoral Care and Education at New York-Presbyterian Hospital; Ms. Trish Sas of The Haworth Press; and Ms. Hee Yung Yi of SmithKline Beecham Pharmaceuticals. Seated at a round table, the guests were important figures in my professional life and especially in my writing of the book. They were from divergent areas, and many did not know one another. So, as Dr. Vandersall described it, "There were many strands that came together that night to make a successful evening."[3] These individual threads were woven into a lovely tapestry that night. I must admit, I was a little anxious prior to this event, as a number of people coming did not know of my blindness. How was I going to handle this event since my celebratory mood was juxtaposed to the others' need to process their reaction to my handicap? God took care of all that. Reverend Hart gave God thanks for the meal, and the rest of the evening was transformed into a wonderful three hours of sharing as if we had all been friends for years. Numerous coincidences were revealed among the guests, most of whom had never met one another before, and that brought the group closer together. In faith, I know these were not coincidences at all but part of God's providence to make this an unforgettable night. Hee Yong Yi told me afterward that there was a real sense of support and pride among the guests for me, for the work I was privileged to do, and for the book I wrote. Debbie Wessely clarified this observation further by saying that people at the dinner, as elsewhere, were impressed by me because I was "able to accomplish so much despite my blindness."[4] Many psychiatrists in the community have told her that they could not do the things I did if they were in a similar position. What people find so striking is the fact that I am not bitter about my handicap. Because I was not born blind, I had to endure a loss. Having lost my vision later in life, many would expect me to be angry, resentful, and preoccupied with my condition. Debbie says that she cannot detect any of that in me. Rather, she observes that I just forge ahead and accomplish goals. People are amazed at this, and I can attribute this only to God. Debbie further described the pride the guests had for me as analogous to when one attends a graduation and witnesses a person who has overcome cancer or some major life struggle to receive his or her diploma. Even if that person is a stranger, many cannot help but shed a tear because they are touched by the situation. Everybody enjoys a good success story! I relate to this, as I have always preferred rooting for the underdog, whether in sports or in life. The evening ended with Mr. Palmer coming to my side and asking if he could give me a hug! This was an unusual request for a person to make in what was supposed to be only a business relationship, but it illustrates well the fellowship tone and easy amicability of that blessed evening. We all had a great time! Since then I have continued to enjoy the strong bond of friendships and professional collaborations with many of those same people.

"SEEK YE FIRST..."

What a wonderful publisher God had found for me. Speaking of finding a publisher, Romans 8:28 states, "And we know that in all things God works for the good of those who love Him, who have been called according to His purpose."[5] Finding a publisher for my book *"Martha, Martha": How Christians Worry* was God's great lesson in my learning to handle rejection. I received multiple rejections from publishers—twenty-one to be exact! I sought out the well-known Christian publishers, as I thought my best audience would be Christians who are interested in psychology and their faith. Tyndale House, Zondervan, Word, Eerdmans, Thomas Nelson, Concordia, Baker, and others were the reputable Christian publishers I sent query letters to over a two-year period. The replies slowly came back, and all showed a common theme—"great idea," "unique book," "interesting content," but "Sorry, mental health and religion are not our marketing needs." In my opinion, this translated to "We do not think this will sell to our readers." God had a different plan. In the summer of 1997, my pastor asked me if I would consider serving in a new counseling ministry at the First Baptist Church of Flushing, a ministry that was being established. I thought, "Oh, no! With all that I am trying to do, why would I want to add another stressor to my already busy life?" However, because of my double training in obstetrics and gynecology and psychiatry, God had given me the experiences needed to serve women who are in crisis when they discover that they are unexpectedly pregnant and contemplating abortion. There was a real need to provide training and leadership in a ministry that helps these women see Christ's perspective in their lives and in the life of the unborn baby. I thought I had better put God first, as it says in Matthew 6:33: "Seek ye first the kingdom of God and all these things shall be added unto you."[6] After much prayer and deliberation, the Lord led me to volunteer at the Boro Pregnancy Counseling Center. For the next year, I devoted all my "extra time" serving on its board and attending to the center's many needs. I had to drop the search for a publisher. Besides, it seemed that I had exhausted the entire list and really had no other Christian publisher to contact. One year later, totally to my surprise, I received a phone call from Reverend Curtis Hart, a hospital chaplain, and the director of Pastoral Care and Education at New York-Presbyterian Hospital. He had just read my article, "Faith and Psychology: Separation or Integration," published in the newest issue of the *Journal of Religion and Health.* He called to compliment me on its boldness and contribution. After thanking him, I lamented that I wished publishers would feel the same way about my book. He asked what it was about and then directed me to try The Haworth Press. The Haworth Press, I learned, was a secular publisher with many book programs, such as business, food, medicine, and international issues. But one of its areas was the religion and mental health book program. This division was well respected and had reviewers who were key thinkers and professionals in the field of psychology and religion. In fact, the book program editor was Dr. Harold Koenig, a well-respected Christian psychiatrist from Duke University Medical Center. The Haworth Press was also highly respected by the North American Association of Christians in Social Work.

By the end of the year, a contract from the publisher was finally in my hands. To my surprise, their market was much larger than I had originally even considered. They dealt with the large national bookstores, Barnes & Noble, Amazon.com, Borders, and others, and many academic libraries and institutions in their active market. This was a miracle I would never have dreamed of. This publisher had the ability to promote to the entire secular trade and academic market, and I had been limiting myself to the Christian market. God must have known that His words written in *Martha* could reach non-Christians as well. In fact, with the recent World Trade Center disaster, I can see the book's role in our society today for the Christian as well as the non-Christian. One day, I was moved to sit down and thank God for each of my twenty-one rejection letters so that I would be directed to His publisher for my book. God's ways are certainly higher than mine, and I ask only that my ways be His.

I was still concerned for the Christian audience. God made a way. Three months after publication, *"Martha, Martha"* was featured prominently on the front cover of The Haworth Press catalog of religious books. This catalog was sent to the entire listing of the Christian Booksellers Association whose membership include the many Christian bookstores in this country—this on top of the large secular market to which they had connections. Praise the Lord for His amazing plans. Although at the time of the publication of the book no one could have ever predicted the events of September 11, 2001, here is how it was used. Barbara Samaan writes:

> The inhumane and horrific terrorist attacks occurring on September 11, 2001, and the prevailing threat of more strikes have generated a heightened sense of anxiety in all Americans. . . . Dr. Elaine Eng's book entitled, *"Martha Martha," How Christians Worry,* is a useful guide in informing and illustrating the different anxiety disorders those survivors and their families may undergo. Moreover, Dr. Eng offers insightful knowledge of how victims' families can support and care for the survivors. In addition, Dr. Eng provides resources that will provide more information and assist the individual(s) in attaining needed professional help. Finally, most importantly, Dr. Eng integrates theological truths with psychological/psychiatric facts by illustrating human apprehension and anxiety through Scripture and God's response to these fears.[7]

The passage from 2 Corinthians 12:7-9 tells me God's grace is sufficient for me and when I am weak, then I am strong. God's strength is made perfect in my weakness. To most of the world, being blind is a weakness and a handicap. Although I realize that there are hardships in having a disability, the positives in view of God's sovereignty far outweigh the negatives. This passage teaches me that as a Christian I can boast in my weakness. I guess I love to testify to God's intervention on behalf of me. I also love to tell the many stories that warm my heart, a type of "chicken soup for the blind." This book is a compilation of many such stories. May the reader find them encouraging, entertaining, and educational in offering insights from the blind perspective.

Chapter 2

Climbing the Wall

On the first New Year's Day of the new millennium, I had the wonderful opportunity to attend a retreat at the Spruce Lake Retreat. The beautiful scenery, fresh air, and sumptuous meals harmonized with the Christian fellowship to restore my entire self. Being blind from my late twenties, you may ask, can a middle-aged woman appreciate the beauty of this idyllic site? With the use of my other senses, I can only heartily say, "Yes, I surely can." There is even more.

On Saturday afternoon, my friend Anna and I chose to take a long hike with Pastor Glen and his family. We wanted to drop in on the nature center and follow it with a walk in the great outdoors. We intended to forgo the other recreational activities scheduled for that time, one of which was climbing the thirty-foot wall located in the gym. This did not seem to be a suitable activity for a blind person, although the idea did intrigue me. In fact, during the week prior to the retreat I had increased exercising my arm muscles in my daily routine, anticipating a possible climb. However, upon arrival at the retreat, I abandoned the idea.

God has never failed to awe me with His amazing plans and strength for the task, whether it is in raising my family, accomplishing professional goals, or even simple day-to-day activities. That Saturday was no different. After returning from our walk earlier than expected, we decided to visit the bookstore. As we made our purchases, Anna exclaimed, "Hey, they're still doing wall climbing!" We entered the gym. As I sat on a chair, I remarked to William, the person sitting next to me, "You know, I think my son was right. I could not climb that wall without sight." William asked, "Elaine, would you like to go up and feel it?" I said that I would. As I approached the wall, I overheard Dave, the instructor, tell someone that he had actually coached a blindfolded person up the wall. In that same instant, I knew that I had to climb it. To the astonishment of the audience as well as myself, I signed up. *What did I get myself into?* I asked myself. Was this utter foolishness, or was there a lesson to be learned from God? I did not have much time to think about this as I was soon being prepped by the instructor for the climb.

> Brothers, I do not consider myself yet to have taken hold of it. But one thing I do: Forgetting what is behind and straining toward what is ahead, I press on toward the goal to win the prize for which God has called me heavenward in Christ Jesus.[1]

This scripture was the best inspiration for the climb. Although it is talking about the attitude one should have about godly effort and perseverance in the Christian walk, it is very analogous to what I experienced climbing the wall. I was determined to scale the wall and strike the bell at its apex. Yet as each muscle strained and I struggled with fatigue, I found that the minutes on the wall seemed like a lifetime. Being blind, I could only feel for the crevices to grab onto; sometimes as I groped there did not seem to be anything within my reach. Only faith in the knowledge that there must be something close by kept my determination strong. The calm, guiding voice of the instructor became my most intense focus. Blocking all other thoughts and distractions, I listened to and trusted his voice to guide me to my goal. What transpired in those moments so much mimics the Christian life. Straining at God's goal for us can at times be fatiguing and frightening and can seem virtually impossible. Yet if you stay focused on His wisdom, strength, and voice, He will help you accomplish what He desires for you. You, in turn, must block out all distractions or negative thoughts. I must admit, there was one moment when I panicked. I was not aware of it, but I was close to the pulley. I heard Dave's voice tensing and telling me I must not grab the pulley, which was connected by a rope to my harness. I was terrified because I did not know how the pulley would feel and how I could distinguish it from the protrusions I was desperately grabbing onto to hold me up. Furthermore,

I had mental images of knocking the rope off the pulley and possibly falling down at least one story. But God was gracious: the back of my left hand gently breezed against something that felt different from the wall protrusions I had been grasping, and I reasoned that this was the pulley I had to avoid. After what seemed to be too many more agonizing stretches, body contortions, and gasping breaths, I heard the glorious sound of the bell as my right hand waved frantically over my head. Hallelujah! What utter joy to know that it is over and done. What relief for my strained muscles as I was lowered to the ground. There is a sense of thankfulness that knows no words or thoughts to accompany it. Rather, it is a very physical, visceral feeling that only my Maker could understand. I will never forget this experience which started off my millennium. It expresses so much of what God has been doing for me in my life and for those whose earnest walk with Him is challenged by disability or struggle.

That night, as I was heading to the cafeteria for dinner, I sensed three large figures—three men—approaching me from the door. A little unsure about the situation, I paused in my tracks. They quickly identified themselves as the director and other administrators of this retreat facility and told me they had heard about how I scaled the wall earlier in the day. Because the camp was used to hosting groups of disabled children sometimes under the leadership of Joni Eareckson Tada, they wondered if they could interview me and write a story on my climb as an encouragement to these children. Of course, I answered, nothing would please me more than to help inspire disabled children to reach their potential. So I agreed to meet their writer and photographer the next day. As I was enjoying a well-deserved and delicious meal with my church friends, our retreat leader came up to me and said the camp director asked if he had a biographical description of me. What kind of request was this? Who carries around a bio? *Wait a minute,* I thought. *Could it be?* Did God, my agent, anticipate this unexpected request? Tucked in my knapsack was a copy of the New Book Announcement I had just received from my publisher. I guess I wanted to show this to my friends from church, so I had packed it. On the second page of this flyer was—you guessed it— a brief bio of the author. I handed this to him, and I think he was as surprised as I was that it worked out so well. So the story of my climb as well as the details of my book went out in the next newsletter of the camp to recipients across the nation. Thanks to God, my agent, the article served as a book promotion in addition to its original intent, which was to encourage those challenged by handicaps.

I believe this is why I wrote, *"Martha, Martha": How Christians Worry.* It is a book about what Christians should know about suffering from anxiety and disorders that cause anxiety. The biblical Martha was a faithful, hospitable believer who was described by Jesus as being "worried and upset."[2] Many Christians suffer for a moment as Martha did, or for days or even months and years. Anxiety disorders are as disabling and challenging as blindness and other physical problems. The book was written as a guide and road map to help sufferers meet the challenge. It comes from my professional work treating many such patients and no doubt from my personal experiences in dealing with the problems of having a visual handicap. In reading the book, people will find ways to get help and be helped. Caring Christians will also find new ways to assist family, friends, and fellow churchgoers who suffer from anxiety. The final message, just like my New Year's experience, is that God makes it possible for all to "climb the wall."

Chapter 3

The Problem with Martha

For with You is the fountain of life; in Your light, we see light.[1]

As a female physician, I have always identified with the biblical figure Martha. She faithfully but busily ran around serving Jesus and others. At times, she even became worried and upset in her activity. But God in His wisdom and mercy told her the benefits of resting at His feet and listening to His illuminating teachings as her sister Mary did.

A premedical curriculum at Princeton University, medical school at the Albert Einstein College of Medicine, and an obstetrics and gynecology residency training at Bellevue and New York University hospitals began my frenzied "Martha" lifestyle. Marriage and the birth of two children, one during my last year of medical school and one during my second year of residency, blessed my life, but certainly created greater demands on my all too limited time. I felt the pain of divided loyalties in wanting to care for my family versus being a conscientious physician who was loyal to her career. Medicine is a strict taskmaster, and women cannot get off the merry-go-round of professional activities easily, but God made a way for me that was totally unexpected.

In 1983, I was diagnosed as having retinitis pigmentosa, an inherited eye disease that would lead to progressive blindness. Once I heard the diagnosis, I knew it was God's way of granting my prayer to be a full-time mom to my babies. God had prepared my heart to accept this news. You can imagine the surprise of my ophthalmologist when I accepted the news enlightened by God's peace. Romans 8:28 says, "And we know that in all things God works for the good of those who love Him, who have been called according to His purpose."[2] This so-called tragedy in my life was very much for the good. I had the chance to "see" and care for my children during their precious young years, to play with them, sing songs, teach them, feed them, and do all those wonderful mothering things that many take for granted. I cherished them because I knew my life was heading in a direction in which I could have missed it all. Now that they are grown, I can see in my mind's eye all of those great images and memories. I enjoyed motherhood so much that I would not have changed my life in any way if given the chance. My eye condition was a gift from God, affording me the privilege of time to be with my children.

I have been questioned about how I can adjust to my blindness without horrendous grief and mourning. I would not have anyone think that blindness is easy. In fact, blind people face many hardships and challenges. To say that coping with these difficulties was pure joy would be a psychological denial of massive proportions. Yet there was a peace and a conviction in my spirit that all would work out well which cannot be explained in human terms or psychological processes. To me, it is a divine intervention—in simple terms, a miracle. It is the grace of God imparted to me to be received by faith. Even the faith I had was given to me as a divine gift, not explicable by any other means known to man. David in the Old Testament may have had the same experience during a time of real distress in his life. He said to God, "You have put gladness in my heart."[3] Somehow this change of heart and mood does not seem to warrant explanation. However, I do apologize to those who cannot fathom the ease of the adjustment. I am bereft of any other words to explain it. I ask that you simply walk with me in my journey and perhaps you will understand.

After my youngest child entered school, I was ready to consider my professional goals again. After much thought, prayer, and advice from Dr. Ed Kong, a Christian colleague and pediatrician, I returned to training in the field of psychiatry. Ed counseled me and said that God would not have taken me through medical school for me to stop now. If psychiatry was the only field in which a blind person could do well, then it must have been God's plan. He also felt there was a great need for psychiatrists who were competent in understanding the faith of their Christian patients. Convinced of this, I applied to hospital residency training programs in psychiatry and was accepted. The transition between the fields of obstetrics and gynecology and psychiatry was quite dramatic. I had not taken even one psychology course in college and did not ever focus on psychiatry in medical school, as that was not my intended area of study. Moreover, the anxiety I now faced in training as a blind physician became daunting. Learning an entirely new body of clinical information and adjusting to the intricacies and challenges of doing it blind would be difficult to say the least. My God was faithful to me. During my residency, objective tests showed that I had started at the bottom and, by the end of the four years, had climbed to the top in terms of psychiatric knowledge. I have now been in practice for many years, working and teaching at the interfaces of psychiatry, obstetrics and gynecology, and Christianity. I believe that the process God took me through in order to accomplish His will in my personal and professional life has taught me much about overcoming disability and the anxiety that can accompany it.

Chapter 4

Heart to Heart

There are many ways to make a good apple pie. You can make a pie with a flaky crust on top or one with a crumb topping. Some pies have raisins in them, and others are plain. Bakers may use different kinds of apples, such as Granny Smith or Macintosh or Golden Delicious. In many ways, the recipe that God uses to make each of us is unique and different. Some of us can be considered tart, some very sweet and sugary, some are a little burnt, and some just plain flaky. Despite our individuality, there is a basic recipe for making a Christian woman, and today I share from my experience, a sort of heart-to-heart discussion.

I am thankful that God would give me the opportunity to communicate my thoughts on women and also their friendships. What makes me the expert? Is it my medical background, my training in obstetrics and gynecology, or the fact that I counsel women? Did I master being a woman of God now that I am middle aged, married for twenty-six years to a Christian man, and have two grown children? Although these are important blessings, I do not think they are what qualifies me. I think what qualifies me are the weaknesses, struggles, and psychological hang-ups I have had that allowed God to use me, teach me, and be my sufficiency as I learned to be a biblical Christian woman.

My background was my first challenge. My mother was born in China—the ninth daughter of a poor family that craved a son. Misled by superstition, they believed that if they gave her up for adoption, their next child would be a boy. So they sold her to a rich, scholarly family who raised her in wealth for a short time, until war broke out in China and she was forced to live in poverty. She grew up feeling that girls were not important. After she married my father and came to the United States, some of her resentment and sadness and also her hopes and dreams as a woman were transmitted to me as her first child, a girl. God had a lot of work to do. Undoing this cultural and psychological heritage was not an easy process. He began by telling me in His Word that He loved me so much that He gave up His only Son to die for me on the cross. Imagine that: I, a girl descended from a family and even a culture that did not favor girls, now had a God who gave up His only Son to die for me. What love. This is the foundation of self-esteem for Christians. Many of us suffer from self-esteem problems that stem from a variety of sources. It could be our upbringing, culture, situations in life, or illnesses. These can prevent us from believing the truth that God tells us about ourselves—namely, that we are created in His image and that He considers us His special children, designated recipients of His absolute grace and kindness. As a psychiatrist, I have seen many Christians suffering from disorders that affect self-image. Depression is an illness that affects people in such a fashion that they do not view themselves positively but rather undergo distortions in their self-image and how worthy of love they feel. They may maintain a false sense of guilt and blame. Anxiety disorders can cause individuals to worry about their adequacies, their futures, or their abilities to function. I try to write and teach about these problems to educate Christians about mental health and psychological issues.

My mother's heritage also brought a second hurdle to my learning to be a woman of God: how to be a submissive woman to my husband, obedient to the biblical teaching in Colossians 3:18, "Wives submit yourselves to your husbands as is fitting unto the Lord."[1] During my entire youth, I pursued the highest academic goals and career plans. I played sports with and against boys with a thirst and a vengeance. It was partly because I loved the competition and partly because I wanted to prove that girls were as good as boys and maybe even better! The Bible does not support this idea, or that one sex is better than the other. We are merely created different. It began to teach me the need for partnership and not competition as a goal in a marriage. With God, I no longer had to prove myself. He loved me as is. All I needed to do was follow His precept for being a godly woman. I praise God for His written standard because it provided a goal for me to accomplish as well as guidance since age sixteen, when I became a Christian. All the psychological and cultural challenges I spoke of I did not understand until my psychiatric training in my thirties. Until then, it was God's Word that kept me accountable to Him while I struggled with my psychological battles. Each of you has inherited such struggles that affect you in different ways. Some you are aware of and some are unconscious, but following God's standard will keep you from the pitfalls of caving into them. Proverbs 31:10-30 provides the best training to be this kind of woman. It set a high standard for me to follow. This was not easy, but by faith I knew that it was worth doing. Peter must have felt the way I did when Jesus told him to cast his net in a certain area. He did not think that he would catch much because he fished there all night with no success. Yet he said in Luke 5 to Jesus, "because you said so, I will do it." He then caught a very large number of fish, enough to fill two boats. That was the way it was with me and the biblical mandate for women. I did not think submissiveness would work for me, a feminist by upbringing, but because God said it, I would try to obey. God gave me great blessings and taught me that His ways were always best. Moreover, I learned that only God could give me the strength to follow His standards. Without Him, I could not possibly do it.

> A wife of noble character who can find? She is worth far more than rubies.
> Her husband has full confidence in her and lacks nothing of value.
> She brings him good, not harm, all the days of her life.
> She selects wool and flax and works with eager hands.
> She is like the merchant ships, bringing her food from afar.
> She gets up while it is still dark; she provides food for her family and portions for her servant girls.
> She considers a field and buys it; out of her earnings she plants a vineyard.
> She sets about her work vigorously; her arms are strong for her tasks.
> She sees that her trading is profitable, and her lamp does not go out at night.

In her hand she holds the distaff and grasps the spindle with her fingers.

She opens her arms to the poor and extends her hands to the needy.

When it snows, she has no fear for her household; for all of them are clothed in scarlet.

She makes coverings for her bed; she is clothed in fine linen and purple.

Her husband is respected at the city gate, where he takes his seat among the elders of the land.

She makes linen garments and sells them, and supplies the merchants with sashes.

She is clothed with strength and dignity; she can laugh at the days to come.

She speaks with wisdom, and faithful instruction is on her tongue.

She watches over the affairs of her household and does not eat the bread of idleness.

Her children arise and call her blessed; her husband also, and he praises her:

Many women do noble things, but you surpass them all.

Charm is deceptive, and beauty is fleeting; but a woman who fears the LORD is to be praised.[2]

Some of you women are single and establishing solid careers given to you by our Lord. Ultimately you have to integrate your professional life with your future marriage and family plans. How do you go from having some autonomy in your profession and then transition into the biblical woman in marriage? The first principle is to accept God's Word as being true and pursue that goal. Look at the Proverbs woman. She worked. She contributed to the household and the material goods of the family. She made real estate and business decisions. She can do all this as long as her attitude is that of love and submission to the authority and the reputation of the husband and love for her family. A Christian woman once told me that she handled the contrast between her high-powered position at work and the submissive role in marriage by a genuine difference in her outward behavior but a consistent inward attitude of allowing God to have sovereignty in both areas of her life. She told me that it worked very easily for her and gave me the courage to think along those lines. It means that women need to exert their authority at the workplace when their jobs require it of them. Exercising authority may be done in obedience to the boss who requires this of you. Ephesians 6:5 supports this by admonishing, "Slaves, obey your earthly masters with respect and fear, and with sincerity of heart, just as you would obey Christ."[3] A woman can honor God in the workplace this way. Even though her husband will not have any influence on her work decisions, he will trust her to make them in a God-honoring way as the Proverbial woman is trusted by her husband. At home, women also have to obey God's word and work in obedient partnership with the husband in managing the home life. That does not mean you agree all the time but that you seek God's will and submit to His plan, taking into serious and prayerful consideration your husband's ideas. Single women can prepare for their future by studying how to be the Proverbs woman. Singles spend much time looking for the right partner, but I think equally important is to prepare to be the right kind of partner for the other person—that is, to prepare to be the kind of woman who will be attractive to the kind of man who values God's standards in a woman.

Once you are married, a couple faces many crossroads. Often, in decision making, there is more than one way of looking at things, and you therefore need to develop an understanding of respecting someone else's perspective and praying to see if God is working out good in their plan. Pray that the spouse's will conforms to God's will and that your will does as well. I constantly pray that my husband exercise good judgment because his decisions will affect me and my children. Remember, he too has a psychological heritage, being the product of his upbringing, culture, and life situations. Sometimes I go along with his decisions even though I disagree and trust that God will work out a better plan for us. That is the blessing of having a powerful God to lean on. You never have to despair that everything will fall apart because of a bad decision on your part or your husband's part. God can make lemonade of lemons if you are His child, called according to His purpose.

Although I am a professional, my most important identity is that of a Christian mother and wife. Because of that important role, I choose to be with women who feel the same. We have a housewife bible study that has been going on for seventeen years. Much of what I learned about being a Christian woman comes from the sharing and lessons I have learned in this group, which has seen more than 100 participants pass through this small but faithful group. We share struggles, our pasts, our unique Asian ways, and even our recipes. We do this all with a commitment to studying and obeying His word. We realize we are not alone. Christian women's groups and friendships teach us that many of our struggles are common—parenting, worries, relationships with husbands, shopping, finances, premenstrual syndrome, and now perimenopause. We also learned that God has the answers sometimes in His word and sometimes from the experiences of the other women. We also know that we can find listening ears and prayerful hearts in such a weekly meeting.

Dr. Irvin D. Yalom, professor emeritus of psychiatry at Stanford University School of Medicine and expert in group psychotherapy, states that group meetings benefit their participants in many ways, including universality, group cohesiveness, support, advice giving, sharing of information, etc. Universality refers to the fact that the group members no longer feel alone or isolated and realize that others have the same issues and struggles. Group cohesiveness gives members a sense of togetherness and belonging, much as a family does. They derive emotional and practical support from one another. Such benefits are being utilized widely in the Christian setting. In 1991, a Gallup study showed that 40 percent of American adults were in a small group which regularly meets. This represents about 3 million small groups. Over one-half of these groups (1.7 million) are church-sponsored adult Sunday or Bible study groups. The rest are secular special-interest groups and self-help groups. The latter may overlap with church groups as certain groups are sponsored by churches. Many of the people surveyed explained that they attend these groups for encouragement, support, a sense of love, and a process in their spiritual journey.[4]

Many women show their love with food. This is especially true in Asian cultures and also in the church. Our Bible study's potluck dishes are legendary as we break bread and share fellowship. In this chapter I share one of my recipes that has been replicated by many women in our group.

No-Brainer Apple Pie

5-7 baking apples
1 frozen pie crust
1 tsp. cinnamon
½ cup brown sugar
¼ cup white granulated sugar
¾ stick butter
¾ cup all-purpose white flour

Peel, core, and cut each apple into eight pieces. Put them directly on the pie crust. Mix cinnamon and brown sugar in a bowl then sprinkle over apples. Cut flour and granulated sugar into butter until crumbly. Sprinkle on top of pie. Bake pie for one hour at 400 degrees. Serve warm or cool.

Now that I shared an all-American recipe, I want you to know that the women have also cooked and shared such dishes as five-spiced braised beef, soy sauce chicken, and noodles made in many different styles. We also have been blessed with international flavors, such as pain bagna, bruschetta, flan, and even stewed caribou. Between the food and mutual sharing we seem to have our own version of Amy Tan's *Joy Luck Club.* I recently saw the movie based on Tan's book which so dramatically portrays the influence of the mother, her culture, and the circumstances of her life on her daughter. These stories are very similar to those I have heard from my own mother; one can see the cultural and personal effects that are passed on. Although the movie focused on the poignant drama of the women's lives and not their Christianity, I do believe God brings about any joy and resolution to their human suffering. God provided the universality and cohesiveness for them to share in one another's tragedy. He orchestrated the reunion of the lost twins with their sister in America. Although the Christian angle was decidedly missing from the movie, it was not absent from my perspective. The friendships among these women were the reason for their ability to overcome great psychological and spiritual burdens.

Women should think about the need for friendship and fellowship with other women. This is important at every stage of life, whether you are a single woman, a wife, or a mother. Some of it will be exciting; much of it will be routine and hard work. Prepare yourselves for it. Choose the company of those who have the same godly values, no matter what stage of life they are experiencing. Plan to be with those who have the fear of the Lord and want to be His instrument—as a woman, wife, or mother.

Chapter 5

Damaged Goods

Six of us sat in a restaurant in the beautiful town of Bar Harbor, Maine. We had just spent the afternoon hiking the two-mile Sand Beach trail at Acadia National Park enjoying the sunny warm weather, salt-scented ocean air, and the incredibly beautiful vistas. My ears were regaled by nature's music played by the regular pattern of undulating waves. My husband and I, along with our dear church friends Tom, Anna, William, and Lucy, were nestled in the relaxing atmosphere on the second floor of Poor Boy's seafood restaurant as the powerful fan cooled us. We in this group make good traveling companions as we enjoy one another's fellowship, friendly humor, and fine food. In fact, these same two couples had accompanied us on a Mediterranean cruise to celebrate our twenty-fifth anniversary the previous year. Having warmed the banks of Rome, Kusadasi (Turkey), and the Greek locations of Santorini, Katakolon, and Piraeus, we now settled on the East Coast of the United States to feast on lobster, spinach lentil soup, broccoli vinaigrette, pasta marinara, fresh bread, and baked potatoes. Of course, some of us had a hankering for Maine's well-known blueberries. So the meal was to be topped off at the end with the restaurant's famous blueberry pie in shortbread walnut crust and vanilla ice cream. Life cannot get any better! Because these folks were like brothers and sisters to me, I took the risk in this idyllic setting to ask a potentially troubling question, hoping not to spoil the mood but to generate good, serious conversation. "Do you think that I could be considered 'damaged goods' to my husband?" I asked, hoping for their thoughtful reflections about how a spouse might view a partner who has developed an unexpected disability after marriage. This was the case with me, as my eye disorder manifested itself about seven years into marriage. Hoping that I would not spoil the evening with such a difficult question, I trusted this small group to be honest and share their comments with the understanding that I wanted to learn about their views and would not take it personally. Neither, I suspected, would my husband, who was listening with interest.

Would a handicapped person be considered damaged goods? Would a diagnosis such as mine cause a spouse to worry about his or her ability to live a normal life or raise children properly? Would he or she be able to handle the dependency needs of the other? What about self-image and how that is jeopardized by being in the companionship of someone who is not physically "whole" or perhaps no longer attractive in the usual media-defined sense? Would the constant stares of strangers in public slowly erode the spouse's sense of self-esteem and thus have an impact on the relationship? Many a marriage has been threatened by illness, not to mention chronic illnesses. When life's storms emerge, many spouses have "jumped ship." Others have held on and weathered the torrent of emotions generated by unpredictability about the future. They negotiate the transitions and the sense of loss, and they make adjustments that are required. I would like to share one of the answers from our dinner table that night that serves as a valuable lesson in life. A parable of sorts, it metaphorically describes my ideal of a spouse's perspective on damaged goods.

A DOG NAMED JADON

Jadon is a young golden retriever, given to my friend's son. It did not take long for this boisterous, affectionate, young puppy to win the heart of my friend, Anna, who referred to him as "our grandchild." Despite his annoying habit of chewing on furniture and shoes, and his sometimes disobedient behavior, he was lovable in so many respects. Daily he anticipated seeing Anna when she returned from work; his ears would perk up and he would dash to her, immediately giving her licks of love. In the morning he would bark his plea for her to feed him and take him for a walk, and she would respond oftentimes as early as 3:00 a.m. Jadon received so much love and attention from his "grandmother" that many a grandchild (even the nonhairy variety) would do well to have even a small portion of this loving attention. There was always a treat for Jadon, whether from the local Petland or even Maine's Bark Harbor. After Jadon was traumatized when a smoke alarm was set off by cooking, he would have the canine equivalent of a panic attack whenever dinner was being cooked. As a result, Anna grilled food upstairs and ordered a lot of take-out in order to keep Jadon calm. This was one truly loved dog.

One day, Anna took Jadon to the veterinarian for his vaccinations. To her surprise, the vet asked, "Did you know your dog is missing a testicle?" Stunned, she answered, "No. The pet store said the puppy was in perfect condition." She wondered what missing a testicle meant. She did not understand what the other one might be doing in the abdomen, as the vet had suggested, or why it was missing. Then she became angry: How could the pet store have sold a dog that was advertised as perfect with such an obvious defect? She felt she had received damaged goods. Then she looked at Jadon and she immediately realized, *I love him. No matter what, I do love him, even if he is not perfect.* The moral of this parable is this: Valued merchandise dissolves the wrath of a cheated consumer. Just like Jadon, I am not damaged goods, at least not to the one who loves me.

My husband has chosen two biblical passages that best express his perspective of me. The first comes from 2 Corinthians 3:2-3, which states: "You yourselves are our letter, written on our hearts, known and read by everybody. You show that you are a letter from Christ, the result of our ministry, written not with ink but with the Spirit of the living God, not on tablets of stone but on tablets of human hearts."[1] He says that I am like a letter written by God for everybody to read—that my life is a testimony to him and those around us and that my blindness serves as a vehicle to provide an encouraging message from God regarding overcoming challenges. I am not a letter written in ink but one written by the Holy Spirit and impressed upon the hearts of people. He also chose Hebrews 12:1-3, which states:

> Therefore, since we are surrounded by such a great cloud of witnesses, let us throw off everything that hinders and the sin that so easily entangles, and let us run with perseverance the race marked

out for us. Let us fix our eyes on Jesus, the author and per-
fecter of our faith, who for the joy set before him endured the
cross, scorning its shame, and sat down at the right hand of
the throne of God. Consider him who endured such opposi-
tion from sinful men, so that you will not grow weary and
lose heart.[2]

This is to say of my life that God is the author of the faith that he
sees in me, a faith that he also possesses and holds dear. Given this
perspective, I have never felt like damaged goods in the presence
of my husband or, for that matter, in the company of those who
love me.

Back to our dinner at Bar Harbor, when I first posed the question about a person being damaged goods, several minutes of discussion and feedback about my blindness followed. Finally, Tom
interrupted with the quip "OK, we've talked enough about Elaine.
Let's get to the point of answering her question about how we feel
about damaged goods. Let's talk about Cliff!" We roared with
laughter, as this comment was so illustrative of the humor and fun
that is essential in coping with disability.

My husband and I had many funny moments as I started to lose
my eyesight. I continue to do most of the cooking, laundry, and
some housecleaning. In fact, I enjoy cooking very much and have
found many ways to do it by choosing recipes that I label as "forgiving" because they can tolerate much error and still taste delicious. I continue to do the chores because I value the sense of independence it gives me. And because repetition makes it easier for
blind persons to retain the ability to do a task, I cherish doing simple tasks of day-to-day living. However, we have had a few mishaps. Watercress is a beautiful green vegetable that makes a delicious soup when it is cooked in a pork broth. Its green color is very
similar to the green scrubbing sponges we keep on our sink to
wash pots and pans. Because they offer no contrast in color to the
watercress, the sponges wound up in the soup one time. As my
husband lifted up the surprise ingredient, he recoiled in horror, and
this has been the subject of many lively evenings recounting to our
friends how his blind wife nearly killed him. Add to that story the
one in which I was removing nail polish with an acetone cotton
ball. I could not find the garbage can, so I dropped it in what I

thought was an empty cup. Instead, it was my husband's Coke. When he went to take the next sip, a strange, chemical odor wafted into his nose and, unfortunately, into his mouth. "Uh-oh," I said. "Well, a little acetone won't hurt you." He also reminds me about the time I used a bath towel to wipe around the kitty litter box and then hung it up instead of discarding it. When he used it to dry his face, he detected a peculiar smell and approached me suspiciously.

Despite these assaults, my husband reacts with good humor to most of these blindness-related incidents, and we both enjoy a good laugh as we entertain our friends with our stories. He wears the black tie-dyed socks and the pink underwear that I inadvertently bleached, thinking I had a full load of whites. He does not seem to mind when his co-workers ask about the interesting patterns on his socks. My children are a little less tolerant, as they have pulled out their ruined outfits from the laundry basket. I guess that is what made them learn to do their own laundry.

After tolerating all these mishaps so well, I have to conclude that I am not damaged goods to my own husband. During our Maine trip, the men were talking a great deal about cars because we needed to buy a new one for our family. A lot of advice was given about consumer reports and which car had the best rating for performance, looks, reliability, and so on. The men enjoyed discussing which was the best model, pointing them out to Cliff as we drove around. Our friends kept insisting that best cars were the Honda Accord, Toyota Avalon, or Nissan Maxima. Again and again they extolled the virtues of these models, and they pretty much had me convinced. My husband—who until this time was barely agreeable to buying a new car rather than choosing a used one, which was his preference—kept saying he really did not want to go with the popular models. He said he would prefer a Saturn. Our friends wanted to know why, as they believed Saturn did not compare with the models everyone else was buying. He said, "I am not like everyone else. In fact, I prefer to choose the different car because it has a different image which better suits me. I like the Saturn because it's different, as I am different. As long as it is reliable!" As his wife, I am like the Saturn—different, not the most popular in the market, but truly reliable in Cliff's eyes. I am a letter of Christ's love, written by God and ordained for my husband.

This reminds me of the hundreds of love letters we exchanged during the years I was away at college and we were dating long distance. Because of our multiple moves and the many years that have intervened, I have unfortunately lost them. It's not so much a tragedy as possibly a mixed blessing, because I would be frustrated by not being able to read them. I certainly would not feel comfortable in having them read to me. So it is better for me to have the memory of them. Besides, the real love letter is written on hearts and not paper or even tablets of stone.

In many ways, God has given me a very suitable life partner. A social worker by profession, he is gratified by helping. When we first got married, I never thought I would become the object of his social work. I also understand him well. My training in psychiatry has helped me to understand his psychological makeup, i.e., why he prefers to be different. Because I understand it, I do not react with disbelief or disdain or take his idiosyncrasies personally. We are a match—slightly damaged perhaps but made in heaven.

THE MOP STORY

Preparing to give a series of talks to an Ambassadors for Christ (AFC) singles conference, I was slightly perturbed by the fact that I was middle aged and somehow too old to appeal to young singles. What did I have in common with them? What could I tell them about womanhood or how to date and find a mate? It had been more than twenty-five years since I went through that process. Moreover, could they relate to me not just because of the stage in life difference, but also in the way I dressed or even the way I looked? My visual handicap could be a barrier and an obstacle in my ability to relate to most people, but especially young people who may not have had much experience dealing with the handicapped. They might therefore feel awkward. God came through again and allayed my worries. I planned three talks—one on managing anxiety, one on womanhood and the Proverbs woman, and one on my personal testimony in Christ. It was after my final talk that a young man wanted to know about my husband. At first I thought he wanted me to address my husband's perspective on being married to a blind person. The young man clarified and said what he really wanted to know was how I met my husband and what attracted me to him. So I recounted the story. When I first became a Christian as a teenager, I attended True Light Lutheran Church. After some time of getting to know everybody, the folks in the church began to talk excitedly about a Clifford Eng, who was coming back from military duty. I kept wondering, *Who is this Clifford Eng who seemed to be friends with all the young people in the church?* One day, I walked into the sanctuary and discovered the answer. There was Clifford Eng mopping the chapel floor. As soon as I saw him, I said to myself, "That's the man for me. He mops and cleans!" After that story, the audience applauded loudly and laughed heartily. The next night at the formal awards dinner, a new award was created for the most godly male single: a brand new mop! During skit night, young men dressed in tuxedos paraded across the stage between acts pushing mops as if in a cleaning frenzy to the amusement of the audience. I hear that my mop story has become part of Ambassadors for Christ singles history.

Chapter 6

Mind the Gap

On the Piccadilly train line running from Heathrow Airport to central London, my son and I were being greeted by the conductor's voice at each stop: "Mind the gap, everyone; mind the gap." Slightly befuddled by the sleep deprivation from our overnight flight from New York to London, we listened with consternation. We were heading for Kenya on a later evening flight and had decided to spend the day in the city, and we were confused by the announcement. What gap are they referring to? Is he asking us to be mindful of such a gap or do we mind that the gap exists? The answer is obvious after one realizes that there is a significant separation between train and platform at each station, and the phrase exhorts passengers to be careful on exiting the train, so as not to get hurt if they put a foot into the gap. The double meaning for me describes the periodic doubts I have about raising my children as a blind mother. Does the now well-adjusted, sleepy young man— sitting next to me on the train because he chose to accompany me on this missionary care trip to Kenya—ever mind the gap caused by his mother's limitations? Is the same young man mindful that his mother cannot do all that other sighted people can do? The same question goes for my daughter, but I will devote the first part of this chapter to my son's reactions. Needless to say, it would be best to ask him his opinion on the matter, but I would like to take the opportunity to free-associate and develop my thoughts on the subject first. So I shall begin by discussing our London excursion.

Our train finally arrived at Piccadilly Circus, which is central to many of London's tourist attractions: Big Ben, Buckingham Palace, Westminster Abbey, St. James's Park, and so on. Camera in hand, Brian escorted me from location to location and I, although not seeing, vicariously enjoyed the fact that he was seeing them for the first time in his life. What surprised me was the fact that he did not seem as excited as I was, and I wondered why. He could be tired since he did not sleep on the flight. He could very well not be interested in London, but he did say he wanted to go. Perhaps it was not a young man's idea of fun to be with his mother on a vacation, albeit only a brief one before going on to mission service. Or could that perennial worry that has crept up in my mind over the years—and more intensely during my children's adolescence—be the case? Are my children ashamed to be seen with a handicapped mother? I know the looks that I get from strangers because many of my friends, colleagues, and family members have described them to me: looks of pity, sorrow, and discomfort. I have always been interested in a full description of others' reactions to me, as human thinking and behavior is my area of study. It is actually quite interesting and fun to observe because it is intellectually stimulating even if not personally experienced. I start to question the opinions of my disability in those relationships that are important to me or when it involves people whose reactions to my blindness may negatively impact my life in some way, whether in job discrimination or unanticipated rejection.

There are times when my doubts are due to my own projection of my thoughts about my handicap onto others. So, are my kids ashamed to be with me at times? To speculate, it probably has happened. It is an honest and human reaction under certain circumstances and in certain stages of development. A teacher once told me that it was lucky I became blind when my children were young, because it is harder when it occurs during their adolescence. I tend to agree with this, as teenagers are quite concerned about self-image and any imperfection may be exaggerated in their minds, including a defect in their parent. Parents of teens are often seen as defective even if they are not so. It is not easy even for the sighted ones. What happens, then, when the parent has a disability? I can speak only for myself. I suppose I could have had my feelings hurt by this extra reason for rejection, but instead it actually prepared me for their adolescence. I had been girded already by the notion that although I had a handicap my identity was not dominated by such an imperfection. I reminded myself that I could not do certain things because I was blind. However, if someone leveled the playing field, I could perhaps do those things through adaptive technology or even with the benefit of having a sighted companion to perform those steps that required sight, and I would follow with whatever it took to accomplish my goal. My life is a challenge because of the handicap, but I am not a handicapped person challenged by life. Having thought this way for many years does gird me for those moments of doubt when I worry that loved ones do not feel the same.

So, Brian and I stopped at many of the major sites of London. By noon, we had worked up an appetite. We were in the mood for Chinese food, possibly a longing for home after many hours of travel, so we started walking in the direction of London's Chinatown. As was the case with the Israelites, we began a wilderness run looking for the promised land of a good restaurant, but we kept going in circles. "Why don't we ask someone?" I asked Brian. "We don't have to," replied my son, "we'll find it." How could he be so sure? When alone, I am used to asking people quite readily from the beginning since, given my limited sight, I have no hope of finding an elusive target. Why waste time? It is not so for sighted people—maybe even less so for men and definitely not so for my son, who continued to lead the way to I-am-not-sure-where. Although I recognized our differences in perspective, it was still hard to be respectful when famished, but we continued on. I wonder how the differences in my perspective have affected my children and whether I have done a good job in conveying that what I do is merely the perspective of a blind person making unique adjustments, but that *my* perspective or behavior does not need to be *their* perspective or behavior. I think of the times when I had to hold the hands of my school-age children just to know that they were safe with me, while other mothers could keep a distant eye on their children and allow them freedom to play. Would I create neurotic children this way? I certainly generated unhappy ones at times when they made me aware that other kids were not holding onto their mothers' hands. I guess I must have relinquished my grip in due time. After all, it is unfathomable to envision holding onto an adult man or woman's hands for his or her safety.

It is amusing to me that although most teens are overly concerned about their friends' evaluations of them, my own children's friends seem to be the greatest supporters of my ability to function. In fact, many of them insist to my own kids that I must be able to see, because I function so well. I guess the consolation prize for having teenagers is the respect of their friends. During those teen years, the parental grass is always greener on the other side—unless that other side has committed a heinous offense.

Happily, the teen years were fairly painless and seemingly short, and our children grew up to be the kind of adults we often prayed for and dreamed about. Brian's college years were very productive. He received a degree in computer science and carried two minors, all in three and one-half years. Beyond that, his college experience taught him leadership in Christian work as he served as a worship leader and president of the Asian-American Christian Fellowship, a campus ministry of InterVarsity Christian Fellowship. One day, he asked if I could speak to this group, at their request, about my experience in publishing *"Martha, Martha": How Christians Worry.* I was shocked, because for years I had the impression that I was incapable of offering to this young man or his peers any possible shred of wisdom. Now they were inviting me to speak. Was he as uncomfortable about this as I was? Was his arm being twisted by his fellow students? Then the doubts flowed. What could I say that would impact the audience and improve my image in my son's eyes? Should I be . . . funny? Serious? Intellectual? Motherly? No, not the latter—that role might be too embarrassing. What was I going to do? Prayer—that's the ticket. At that point I needed nothing less than divine intervention, and that's what I received.

I walked into their storefront meeting place and was greeted by a group of college students, some quite friendly and others shy and retiring. Without sight, only the former are recognized easily. The others are lost to perception unless they pipe up later. The leaders gathered together to pray for me and for the night. Then God worked His magic. By the time it was done, the students were really engaged, entertained, and encouraged. I had a lot of fun, and my books were selling like review manuals at finals time. Brian told me he thought it went really well, which was the best reward I could have had. The Lord had used him to be my agent in the college world, and it was a success. I should have known that it was not the risky business I feared it would be, but that is where my faith will have to grow.

RED SHOES
AND THE "BLIND NEUROTIC THING"

My son's reply to the query, "What is it like having a blind mother?" was somewhat different from my speculations. Most of his complaints of me as a mother are the usual things that mothers do—I always think I am right; I treat him like a child. Regarding the blindness, he says that because he has been living with my blindness since he could remember, he does not feel he has missed anything due to my limitations. He seems to think that I carry on pretty much as any mother would. However, he does have complaints because of my blindness, which both children will heartily articulate—my choice of clothes and how I match—or rather do not match—them. Their biggest source of horror is my pair of red shoes, or more specifically, a pair of bright red Reebok high-top sneakers I inherited from a friend. I have put on this most comfortable pair of footwear with, I guess, the most outlandish combinations of clothing, including my green down coat, a tank top with a tropical medley of orange and blue flowers, and pink sweatpants. To me, if the clothes feel good, they ought to look good, but the rational side of my mind tells me and, more important, my children tell me that this is not so! My daughter insisted that she pick out my outfit for her high school graduation. I gladly assented, as I certainly wanted to make her day as smooth and pleasant as possible. Besides, I hate shopping and choosing my clothing. The only garments that appeal to my blunted vision are usually in the gold-and-black combinations which wind up as fabric usually meant for an upholstered couch and not women's wear. The only relatively safe colors I can buy are all-black or all-white items, which require no effort to match to other items as they will almost always "go." It is funny, because I do defer to my family in choosing my clothing, and especially to my daughter. So there was a time when Gen was about five to eight years old when I wore a lot of pink frills. Then I went through a black phase during her adolescence. Happily, she is in her twenties now and it will not be long before I will dress appropriately for my age. I thank God for classic business suits as they keep me from utter ridicule during office hours or when speaking in front of people!

They have another complaint of their blind mother that all three of us call the "blind neurotic thing." Its origins are probably that I am somewhat neurotic to begin with; they say you have to be in order to become a physician. This is accentuated by the addition of a handicap. For example, I insist on having things done my way because I think that I am correct even when I am not. A recent conversation about purchasing a new family car that is safe and sturdy led me to insist to my kids that Volkswagen Beetles are not safe. To my recollection, these "bugs" look like a can of peanuts waiting to be opened by the slightest impact. Of course, I have not seen a VW in twenty years and was told that they no longer look like my mental picture of a VW. What irks my children is that I can be so emphatic based on old (to them) facts. I have to say in my defense that my image of them feels very current. My picture of the present is composed of images I saw decades ago. The positive side of this is that, to my mind, neither my husband nor I have aged. What a blessing, as I do not fret over our looks as many of our middle-age peers do. Back to my children and this "blind neurotic thing": the car conversation does not compare with the genuinely upset feelings generated by the following anecdote.

My son's church basketball team was in a heated, neck-and-neck competition in a summer tournament. They were counting on winning the next game to place first, and Brian was one of their key players. However, earlier that month I received a frightening phone call that Brian had been cut in the eye during basketball and would have to be taken to the hospital. My husband and I hurried to the emergency room with thoughts too unimaginable to articulate. Fortunately, Brian's laceration was just above his eye and not to the eye itself. It was sutured by a plastic surgeon. Brian was admonished by the doctor not to play ball or do anything that might reopen the wound in his eye area. Now, a month later, his friends were pleading with him to help win the game. Although torn by their dilemma, I insisted that he could not play based on his doctor's recommendation and my fear of having him hurt the wound again. Needless to say, he was quite upset that I did not even consider his assessment of being well enough to play. His friends pleaded with me to let him play, but I held my ground with an unusual determination, which was quite uncharacteristic of me. It was not until after a year of enduring his lingering hostility about this event that we discussed it, and I then realized that part of my unrelenting stance was because the injury had something to do with his eye. My irrational fear was that he might have been blinded. I had the intuitive feeling that I was quite traumatized at the time of his injury but assumed it was a usual maternal reaction. Only my composed doctorly self kept me matter of fact during his treatment in the emergency room. In discussing it with Brian, I recognized that as much as I thought I had adjusted to blindness, I could not bear the thought of it afflicting my children. So this is what we call the "blind neurotic thing," and I hope to be able to recognize this in myself in the future. It might help me let go in those instances that I should. Thankfully, retinitis pigmentosa has the kind of recessive inheritance pattern in which it should not affect my children unless my husband also unknowingly carried the gene. This revelation also reminded me of when my daughter was in second grade and she said she had trouble reading because her vision was blurred. Rather than taking her to the regular optometrist, I proceeded directly to the top pediatric neuropthalmologist in the area—talk about overkill. Somehow I needed to be reassured that her sight was not affected as mine was. So when I got the news that children often get blurry vision when tired, I was relieved. All that she needed was temporary reading glasses from the drugstore if she had the symptoms again. Later she confessed to me that the only reason she complained of blurred vision was that she wanted glasses like her friends had. It serves her right that we bought the cheapest, ugliest pair available at that drugstore. This is the same child who told me she had taken her erythromycin for her strep throat even though I found the big pink pill in the kitchen garbage can. I guess they think they can pull fast ones on their blind mother, but a mother's intuition and knowledge of her children can make up for a lot of visual deficits!

MEMORIES AND FANTASIES

"Your mother is a CIA agent," my daughter's college friend Nick told her. "She functions too well to be really blind. I'll bet all that traveling she does to give talks is really undercover missions she does, posing as a blind person!" Nick and I met only briefly when he spent part of his summer vacation with our family. How he came up with this idea probably had very little to do with our meeting but had a lot to do with my daughter's accounts of my work to her friends. She is pretty clear in stating that "my blind mother can do more than many that are sighted." Although I cherish the fact that she seems proud of me, I suspect she must embellish the story a bit. In any case, God deserves the credit, lest I develop a swelled head. With her stories about her mom, Genevieve cannot convince new friends that her mother is blind. Even in high school, one of her best friends, Peter, insisted that I was not at all blind but was into the charade for the blue handicap sticker that allows us to park our car in privileged spots. He spoke of our family as picture perfect, living in a house with the proverbial white picket fence. Although humorous to me, who cannot even see my beige, fenceless, Tudor home, I appreciate the image conveyed. Where else but in the mind of an imaginative Korean teenager could we get an all-American snapshot of the perfect family that includes a married couple with one son and one daughter, where the mother is posed in her dark glasses and white cane? All-American family indeed!

Let me share my memories about first getting the cane. For years after my diagnosis was made, I hesitated to obtain a cane. It was partly because I did not think I needed it, since not all of my vision had deteriorated, and partly because getting a cane would call attention to my handicap. Using the cane would give me an instant new identity to others and highlight to myself that I was a blind person who needed to adjust to others' reactions to me, including the reactions of strangers. I was not ready for it until one day, when crossing the street, I almost got hit by a bus because I did not see it. The driver probably figured I saw him and therefore should have moved more quickly, like most New Yorkers would.

Little did he know that I was not like most New Yorkers, nor did I give him any clue or warning to slow down. A mobility trainer taught me how to use the cane to feel and make a clear path for myself as I walked. There is a rhythm to the sweeping motion, back and forth, that is matched by the cadence of one's gait. Everything is precise in order to ensure safety, automaticity, and consistency in its use. Any veering from the rules in which I was trained often led to accidents. Before long, the pain of such injuries reminded me never to slack off in its proper use. It truly opened up my world, as I found I could travel farther on my own when walking in my neighborhood. Shortly after mastering the cane, I started my residency training in psychiatry. My fellow residents laughed with me as we found that in the hospital, getting to the cafeteria for lunch would be much faster if they put me in front to clear the path through the crowds with my sweeping cane. I think a good sense of humor helps to dissipate any discomfort among others. Once, I met with a senior resident for the first time to get adjusted to being on call in the hospital. Somehow, my cane picked up something from the floor that stuck to it and it dragged along down the halls as we walked. When I realized what happened, I remarked that this special cane had the dual purpose to not only guide me but also to pick up garbage at the same time. Corny as the joke was, he laughed loudly, partly because of the humor but mostly at the relief that I can joke about my dependency on it. Most fascinating was the reaction of my church friends. Although three years earlier we had told them about my diagnosis and the prognosis of eventual blindness, they did not fully react until the day they saw me for the first time walking up to the altar for communion with my white cane. My husband got many remarks and questions that day. They all asked something to the effect of "She really isn't *that blind,* is she?" I guess there comes a time when psychological denial no longer works, and nothing helps to overcome it like the traditional white cane.

Children have a fascination for the cane. I often hear the young voices in the bank or supermarket asking their mothers in loud unabashed voices, "Mommy, what's that stick for?" Sometimes their mothers explain its purpose in matter-of-fact detail, but many would try to hush their children and move them to a distant place before venturing an explanation, as if they might hurt my feelings if they explained it within my earshot. Young children relate to handicapped persons quite well until they are taught to be uncomfortable. I have been entertained by young ones whom I have befriended that ask if they can borrow my cane to help them walk. It is as funny as the many times my young daughter would find a wooden stick and use it just as I used my cane when she walked with me. It is very funny for others to see a tiny girl with big sunglasses holding a small tree branch and swinging it from side to side. Of course, she stopped this behavior as a teenager. Today, this childlike identification has been taken over by my four-year-old niece, who proudly walks with my cane.

LESSONS IN FAITH

What can I, as a mother, teach my children through my experience with the challenges of blindness? I am in some ways a shepherd to my family, a teacher, a role model, as well as a mother. As with any group I mentor, encourage, or inspire, I do not want only to entertain them with stories about my life but hope to instill lessons applicable to their own lives. Here are the lessons in faith I have learned.

How does that little girl with the oversized sunglasses and the wooden cane that she does not really need walk? For that matter, how does her blind mother with the real white cane get from one place to another? By putting one foot in front of the other and repeating the process: left foot, right foot, left foot, right foot . . . Although this seems trite, it is not at all simple. There are many things involved. But the key is faith, and more explicitly, *trust.* One must have a lot of trust to walk. First, you must trust the cane to tell you that the path in front of you is indeed clear. Then you must trust that the direction that you are heading in is the correct one, or you will be wasting time and probably get lost. Worrying about this will cause you to hesitate to go forward. You may also have to trust the person or persons who come to your assistance at any point in your travels. Many times you need to make decisions as to whether you can trust any of these things, and you could, at any point, doubt the trustworthiness of them all. Trust requires thinking and assessment; an educated sense of human nature; teachability so that you can learn from your mistakes; and an ability to remember all those things and people on whom you can rely. Yet all this is not enough. At any point along the road, you can be paralyzed. Disorientation from untrustworthy cues, a loss of faith in the cane when you have tripped over a crevice it missed, or a lack of a person to assist you when you are at some confusing crossroad—all can halt any progress you have made. What, then, is required to ensure progress, whether in traveling or in life? My only answer and what has worked for me is the absolute faith in God; I trust Him and believe He is supervising my entire adventure. The knowledge that He sees what is going on, even though I do not, is enough to reassure me that I can put my left foot in front of my right foot and go on. Sometimes in a moment of nagging fear, I recall the hymn, "Guide Me, O Thou Great Jehovah"[1] and walk to the rhythm of the melody. Soon all fear and doubt are diminished by the tones of the song and the message it conveys. Or I think about the angels that God employs to protect His children and I am reminded that "I know that there are angels all around" me, a line from another song.[2] Somehow the content of these two thoughts work to remind me that I am safe in my travels with a sovereign God watching over me and allowing me to make progress from point A to point B. I mean this both literally as I walk about and also figuratively as I negotiate my personal and professional life. As the verse says, "We walk by faith . . ." The Bible continues with ". . . not by sight."[3] Then, how is a blind person to "see"?

Heavenly vision is my definition of what faith allows me to see. It takes on many forms, but clearly its source is the Lord. How many times have I lost something and have asked God to put me right in front of that item, since I have no other way of locating it when alone. Within a short time, the object would be in my hands, to my surprise, at least initially. Now with repeated occurrences, I am no longer surprised but am still very thankful. Trying to teach this spiritual concept to a sighted person looking for something is like teaching a gourmet chef how to open a can. It is preposterously simple and often deemed by the individual to be unnecessary, but strand him or her on a desert island with only wood for kindling, a can opener, and some canned goods, and he or she will take on a different vision. My eye condition puts me in a similar position, and I have discovered the perspective that a simple trust in God is vital no matter how much one thinks one owns or possesses!

Heavenly vision also refers to those cues I get that help to gain insight into a situation or a person that others obtain from their eyesight. Some people cannot even identify certain insights despite their eyesight, or perhaps their vision may mislead them. Call these heavenly insights intuition, but I believe they can be broken down into the following components. I refer to cues from our surroundings that do not require vision.

Sound

It is amazing how much one can tell about a person's mood by listening to the tone and tension in his or her voice, as well as by paying careful attention to what is being said. It really does not take a rocket scientist to know how a person is doing by carefully listening. Yet in our visually dependent, overstimulated, and rushed lives, we do not take the time to develop our listening skills.

Scent

Scent is still another cue. Favorite perfumes, soaps, or deodorants have often helped me identify a person as he or she walks into a room. Odors and the lack of such perfumes can tell me whether a person is ill, depressed, or too busy to take care of himself or herself. All of these can be addressed as I serve my family, my friends, or my patients. Many have asked me if my other senses became sharper when I became blind. The answer is yes and no. I do not believe they got sharper, but I have gotten much better at using them since I have to rely on them more often. For example, I can always rely on my sense of touch to pick the best fruits and vegetables in a grocery store. Add to this the smell of ripeness and it is a cinch to obtain perfect produce.

Wisdom

Heavenly vision also has a lot to do with wisdom, and by this I mean the wisdom and truth that are found in the Bible. You get so many versions of the truth as you listen to others describe it to you from their perspective. Therefore, I need an anchor, and for me the time-honored, well-used, blessed word of God becomes my choice when I need to "see the light." It is such a great source of heavenly insight, and my ability to trust in it has fueled the way for many of the accomplishments of my life. Without it, I would be fearful even to proceed.

God's Insight

Finally, heavenly vision does include an indefinable aspect, what I could only describe as God's provision of insight from His resources, other than those I have just described. When all the known tangibles are factored out, there is the large category of things you see because God has put the conviction and vision in your spirit. When this happens, I trust this as if it were sight. It is then confirmed by many circumstances. When I reach my destination or goal, there is great rejoicing in my heart that His vision is not only trustworthy but also realizable!

The third faith lesson I want to pass onto my children from my experiences is that we must live by faith. Psalm 127:1 says, "Unless the Lord builds the house, its builders labor in vain. Unless the Lord watches over the city, the watchmen stand guard in vain."[4] This verse teaches that faith in God must be the foundation of a person's marriage, family, vocation, ministry, and security. I have been blessed by His presence and orchestration of all these aspects of my life. Do not get me wrong; I am not perfect in all these areas, since at times I try to take control over one or all of these spheres of life, despite my knowledge and determination to let God rule. Yet my determination to have Him be the foundation for my personal and professional life has always been my deepest desire, and God has honored my intention with His grace and help. My marriage, family, vocation, and ministry have given me deep satisfaction and joy—so much so that I have no regrets in any of these. What about security? Can I stand safe and secure in all these things I have listed? Psalm 127 tells us that the sighted watchmen stand in vain to guard the city if the Lord is not watching over it. This answers the question. The blind person whose foundation is God has infinitely more security than the sighted, knowing that the Lord is watching over his or her domain. I have full trust in this fact and therefore remain secure. This security is a priceless treasure, and I believe it is what prompts me to keep persevering with joy in the Christian life. God has taught me such valuable lessons in faith in my disability. Truly He is able to help overcome any challenge in life. May my children be blessed with this legacy, and may I continue to model it as I shepherd them along.

Chapter 7

A Mentor for Women

Likewise, exhort older women to be in the manner of life reverent, not slanderous, not having been enslaved to much wine, teacher of what is good, so that they may train younger women to be loving their husbands, loving their children, self-controlled, pure, working at home, being kind, being subject to their own husbands in order that the word of God may not be blasphemed."[1]

Barbara Samaan, a pastor's wife who is blessed with the gifts of leadership and encouragement, enjoyed her ministry to women. An effective mentor especially to young adult women, she is instrumental in shaping their Christian lives. She has a genuine concern for discipleship, prayer, and developing a strong relationship with these women through which she openly shares how God has molded her in her own journey. As a pastor's wife, Barbara is exposed to many situations requiring counseling, and she is often called to intervene in crises. Sometimes the work can be quite draining and other times she finds herself very capable and effective in her work. She feels the key to success is to have a strong relationship with God, a solid quiet time with Him in prayer, and meditation on the Word each day. She says if she does not start with that, the day's work is "shot." Her spiritual gifts, role in the church, and personality lend themselves very much to the successful mentoring of women. When asked about her own mentoring needs, Barbara confesses that there are only a few mentors in her life. She does find her husband to be a valuable resource.

Christian books and tapes provide much information and insight for her, and she devours them eagerly. She then likes to dispense her insights from them to those she mentors. Although books are not really human relationships as mentors are, they do serve a purpose in informing and confirming. I remember that at a funeral we bumped into each other and she asked me if I could please go to her church and talk about *"Martha, Martha": How Christians Worry*. I was touched by the kind request, as I was relatively inexperienced at being an author. This was one of the earlier invitations I had received and since then have received many more from Barbara and her church. She later explained to me that, because I was a psychiatrist and a Christian, it impressed her as to what I was capable of doing. Also, the situations that require her to do counseling in her church are similar to those I handle in my practice. She feels that I am qualified to provide information and guidance to her and those in her position. When I asked her how she felt about my sightlessness, she said, "It was not at all an issue, partially because you never let it become one. I was drawn to your abilities as a professional and never felt that the blindness was a hindrance or a consideration."[2] I tried to elicit more feedback from her, because it was hard to believe that my blindness was never an issue and perhaps she was just being kind or, as many do, she was denying the presence of my handicap. However, I realized soon that she genuinely did not find it to be a problem. She sees that I negotiate obstacles with resourcefulness and get help when needed, yet the blindness is not my main preoccupation, but rather it is the tasks or goals at hand. We have enjoyed a wonderful relationship planning a women's conference and doing programs at her church, and she has turned out to be one of the many that God has used to be my agent.

Barbara's leadership also comes out in her nurturing, motherly style, which suits her well. It is reflected not only in her discipleship of women but also in her cooking. She often cooks for large groups and has some awesome recipes for large gatherings. I told her about recipes that I use which are very forgiving—that is, they come out well even if you do not see what you are putting in. I often use my hands to measure ingredients into a pot or a bowl, and therefore there is often variation in the amounts used, but forgiving recipes come out great anyway. One night I offered to cook for twenty-two people from the setup crew for a comedy program done by the "Clean Comedians" called "Laugh for Life." Barbara supervised me as I cooked two of her own forgiving recipes, which were delicious! Even the comedian had only good things to say about the meal, although I was half-hoping for some funny jokes about a blind person cooking for a crowd. My hungry guests had a merry time eating and sharing fellowship with one another before the show. A true "chicken soup for the blind" moment. Included in this chapter are the two recipes I used from Barbara's collection.

Chicken and Rice

6 lbs. chicken parts (drumsticks and thighs are good)
4 cups uncooked rice
6 cups water
2 cans cream of mushroom soup
2 cans cream of chicken soup
2 envelopes Lipton onion soup mix

Mix all ingredients together except the chicken and put in large aluminum pan (18 inches x 11 inches). Put chicken pieces on top of mixture and push them down to sink into mixture. Seal pan tightly with aluminum foil or lid. Bake for 2 ½ to 3 hours at 350 degrees. Make sure rice is soft by lifting foil and checking at corners of the pan.

Hamburger Goulash

3 lbs. ground beef or turkey
3 lbs. cooked elbow macaroni
6 cans tomato soup
3 cups grated American cheese (can substitute 1 8-oz. can of Parmesan cheese)
1 tsp. salt
½ tsp. black pepper

Cook and drain meat. Add elbow macaroni, soup, and some of the cheese, reserving ½ cup to the side. Mix all ingredients and stir briefly on low heat until cheese is melted. Sprinkle with remaining cheese.

What does Barbara teach us about the biblical role of mentoring? First, Titus provides instruction to the early believers in Crete to lead lives reflective of godly behavior. In this book, which defines proper Christian behavior to older and younger men, slaves, and women, the admonition is for older women to live reverently, not to be slanderous or enslaved to wine. Rather, as examples of godly behavior, they should teach younger women to love their husbands and children, attend to the home, be kind to those in the household, be self-controlled and pure, and subject to their husbands. This is done in order that the gospel of God not be blasphemed. In other words, godly behavior on the part of all, but especially in the mentoring of women, is done so that the witness to the world of the Christian life remains pure and not ridiculed in the eyes of the nonbeliever.

Chapter 8

The Navajo Experience

Fay is a soft-spoken, godly woman who has served on short-term missions to the Navajo people almost every year for the past eleven years. She enjoyed watching her three daughters grow and mature from this experience and gain responsibility in caring for others, especially the Navajo children. She states that they have developed from very young children to mature, dependable teen-agers without her telling them what to do. She has learned a great deal about other people, including the Navajo and their cultural differences, as well as about her missionary teammates. In fact, she has learned much about herself in the process. She states she was very naive about people and spiritual issues prior to her trips but has acquired wisdom in the process.

In 1996, my son and I had the opportunity to do a short-term missionary trip to the Navajo reservation in Hard Rock, Arizona, under Fay's leadership. A group of twenty-two people from vari-ous churches joined together, and, after months of training and preparation, ventured up to Little Black Spot Mountain where Mattie, a Navajo Christian woman, and the Courtneys, a mission-ary couple, invited us to help them with their work. Much of our team's efforts were divided between doing labor projects at the compound and doing vacation Bible school for the Navajo chil-dren. I was asked to help teach the adults, but when I learned that the Navajo-speaking teacher was not going to be there that sum-mer, I wondered how I was going to communicate with the non-English-speaking adults. My coteacher, a seasoned member of this project, did not seem too disturbed, so I decided I was not going to worry about it. Instead, I would diligently prepare my lessons and then keep an open mind as to how they would be taught. It is quite a challenge to connect without language, and then, in my case, without the visual cues to help with pointing, basic sign language, or even a way to detect facial expressions. On what level could I relate to the Yazzies, Grandpa Goy, Mattie, and the older women? I knew that the Navajo very much enjoyed crafts and working with their hands. In fact, they are renowned for some of the finest wool rugs in North America. According to legend, their weaving skills, a tradition passed on from generation to generation, was said to have been taught by the spider. This spider was deified by the Navajo and called "the holy spider woman." Their rugs, I learned, were a highly desirable art form. They had an ample supply of wool obtained from raising sheep for food as well as for clothing. Although I had no hope of using any kind of loom, I knew that with my fingers I could do simple crafts by touch. I thought perhaps we could communicate and have a relationship in working side by side making crafts together and then I would go on from there. I found myself putting the wood and plastic pieces together of a *gna-lookie* (Navajo for "butterfly"), as a group of my students bemusedly helped their blind teacher. I'm not sure whether they were chuckling at my inept crafting skills or the funny way I kept saying *gna-lookie* to improve my pronunciation. No matter what, the bond was created, and I found I enjoyed this company of people, so different yet so similar, who maybe even shared common ancestors from the continent of Asia. Thankfully, there was an excellent translator in my class, the daughter of a Navajo convert to Christianity, and she made the actual teaching quite simple. I did request that most biblical readings be done in Navajo, because I think students get more out of a class if the primary language is their own. Besides, I cherish hearing scripture in other languages because it reminds me that my faith is universal and not a product of my own culture or mind-set.

The Navajo are a matriarchal society, and much of the socialization and child rearing is in the hands of the women. The woman is the shepherd, farmer, businessperson, ruler, and meal planner. The food is wholesome and inexpensive as a rule. Mutton is the primary meat used, and I truly enjoyed their mutton stew with hominy (dried corn). This was accompanied by our simple cuisine of spaghetti, instant Chinese noodles, and sandwiches that we hurriedly shopped for at the big warehouse supermarket while driving from the airport to the reservation. Our mission team were no worse off in our "limited" menu. In fact, I dare say many of us gained weight. Oh, the hardships of mission life. I have included one recipe that we learned from the Navajo women, called Navajo Fry Bread.

Navajo Fry Bread

1 cup white flour
½ tsp. salt
¼ cup powdered milk
1 tsp. baking powder
½ cup warm milk
Shortening to cover ½ inch of a skillet when melted (can substitute oil)

Mix ingredients and knead gently to form a soft dough. You may have to add small amounts of water gradually to make the dough consistency soft. Place dough in bowl and cover with a cloth for one hour. Shape dough into tennis-sized balls and flatten into eight-inch rounds. In a pan of hot shortening, place circle of dough flat on the pan and fry for two minutes on each side until golden brown. Use medium heat, but watch carefully that the dough does not burn. With a fork, pierce any bubbles that may form in the dough while it is frying. Drain on paper towels. Serve with honey or use as soft tacos for chili or other fillings. You may also use chopped tomatoes, lettuce, and cheese as a filling. You may also pan-fry on a nonstick pan without using shortening.

Caring for the children was a tiring but gratifying task for many of our team members. The children are an active, boisterous group, unlike the quieter adults. They were always so happy to see the Chinese team come to their community. Each year a team composed of representatives of the Chinese-American churches in New York would come to teach vacation Bible school (VBS). The Navajo children would herald our arrival with the cry, "The Chinese are coming!" Many of the older kids loved to play basketball with the team. The Navajo youngsters, and especially the young women, prided themselves on their ball-playing skills, often winning awards for their schools. Although I could not see them, I can tell from the noise that the children enjoyed our stay. At times, I would feel a little wistful and perhaps useless as I really could not join in the activity. However, my inertia was often subtly interrupted when a missionary or a teammate would ask to speak to me for some advice or counsel. It took quite a long time and several missions trips before I realized that this was my special role in the field, and that instead of longing to be part of the main activities I needed to be available on the sidelines so that the other missionaries could have a person to speak to. I later learned that what I was doing was part of what is called "missionary care" or "member care." How dense could I be? Instead of wishing I could wave these people off and do real work, God was saying this *is* your work! This highlights a very important aspect of missions and life in general: teamwork. In the microcosm of the Navajo experience, I learned the importance of recognizing that each person had a different gift, talent, or predisposition to offer the group. No one person is more needed than another. "Sam," the missionary in charge of maintenance, said it best in his chapel sermon: "We work as an ensemble. And in an ensemble, there are no stars." Rather, the persons making up an orchestral team ideally labor in a harmonious way, each instrument contributing to the quality of the music.

A comical skit done at the evening fellowship gathering also demonstrated this point. I acted as the woman who needed to get dressed for a big event, when suddenly all my clothes (portrayed by other actresses on the team) popped out of my closet. Each item of clothing argued that it was the most beautiful, most essential, or most logical and should be worn. These clothing items got into a real scuffle, to the laughter of the audience, and it was finally broken up by my embracing but firm biblical statement that they were all necessary, each serving a different purpose in my wardrobe, just as each person has a role in the body of Christ. Oscar-winning actors we were not, but the wisdom of our message prevailed. Our entire team was joined by the attitude of being an ensemble.

As a blind person, I have always found it easier to feel accepted and productive in the church or in the company of people united in ministry. It is precisely because of this notion of the body of Christ being composed of different parts, each with unique qualities and roles, that contributes to a greater whole. Even those parts that the rest of society may not deem useful or that may be considered a burden are valuable in the eyes of God. This directly challenges the fear that most disabled persons maintain; that is, they are no longer useful because they are not able to do what they once did and are now dependent on others. The biblical perspective says that dependency is not always bad; in fact, it is needed in the body model, and that despite disability, God has designed and even ordained a special place and role for the disabled. This truth has always kept me on a positive track in my work and in my church life. It is especially therapeutic if, in the course of things, frustration or doubt gets me discouraged. I try to "see" things from this heavenly perspective and "look" for the purposes and roles I am to take. When searching for such, they often appear to me in abundance. This perspective is not always easy to maintain, but its truth is essential. Perhaps being visually blind can facilitate this perspective; at least it did for me. It follows the Bible verse: "While we look not at the things which are seen, but at the things which are not seen: for the things which are seen are temporal; but the things which are not seen are eternal."[1] Teamwork—and in particular, God-directed teamwork—is an important means of coping for the blind individual, and the Navajo experience highlighted that for me.

Our group took one day off to visit Canyon de Chelly in Arizona, not far from Little Black Spot Mountain, where we were staying. It was the typical sunny, hot, dry, 100-degree-plus Southwestern day, as we drove off intending to make the three-mile hike down and then up the canyon. The hairpin turns on the mountainous trail down were daunting for those who could see the drop-off at each cliff. The return climb was less scary but much more exhausting. It was quite a challenge as I clung to the elbow of Pastor Howard to make the descent and ascent. Besides being able to say one did this feat, what truths could one learn? First, I learned to have a real appreciation for water. Constantly, our team had to make rest stops and replenish our bodies with the bottled water we carried. It is so reminiscent of the psalmist's words, "As the hart panteth after the water brooks, so panteth my soul after thee, O

God."[2] Recognizing the need for spiritual water as well as physical water is adaptive in life, especially in taxing times. What helped me most, especially in the final leg when I had no more strength, were the words of the children's song, "One step at a time, I'm climbing that mountain, one step at a time with Jesus at my side."[3] In order to get somewhere on an arduous road, one can only think about it as one step at a time. If you start worrying about the entire trip and what difficulties may befall you, you may be so discouraged that you are prevented from proceeding. So it is with my journey with blindness. It has always been one step or hurdle at a time. With each successful step, I get the encouragement to take the next, as long as Jesus is at my side.

It's only fitting that I close this chapter with the Navajo translation of the popular Christian song.

Baa ha'niih, baa ha'niih, baa ha'niih, baa ha'niihgo Boholniihii Bo – hol – nii – hii ei baa ha'niih![4]

Hallelu, Hallelu, praise ye the Lord, indeed!

Chapter 9

A Trip to Mexico

I will lead the blind by ways they have not known, along unfamiliar paths I will guide them; I will turn the darkness into
light before them and make the rough places smooth. These
are the things I will do; I will not forsake them.[1]

On a Sunday morning, as I was walking from the parking lot to
Chinese Evangel Mission Church, I felt an intense desire to go
serve the Lord in a Spanish-speaking country. That was strange, I
mused. There was no rational motive or forethought for this com-
pulsion. That very same Sunday, the announcement was made
about a short-term mission project in Mexico being planned by Dr.
Anthony Wong. A shudder passed through me as I recognized that
what I had experienced in the parking lot was most likely a calling
from God. So, to confirm my suspicions, my daughter, who revealed that she was considering going to Mexico as well, became
my "Gideon's fleece." I prayed that God would convince her of His
will. If she was led to participate, that would be my confirmation
to serve as well. And God said, "Go."

Three Reasons for Going

Amid the many trials, anticipatory anxiety, and oppressive events
prior to departure, it was vital to cloak the entire venture in prayer.
The experience of preparation for this trip was decidedly unpleas-
ant. First, I had to grieve the fact that I could no longer provide the
primary medical care that I cherished doing when I was in obstetrics and gynecology. I knew I would be in a place where there was
the need for this type of medicine, and that I could no longer do it
because I had developed a condition that caused blindness. This

mission project would be a psychological reminder of my professional angst. I would reexperience my loss anew each time I could not help a woman with a gynecological need. In addition, my mother's diagnosis of breast cancer the month before my trip created a further sense of helplessness, which is most disturbing to the emotional life of many physicians. More obstacles arose in the preparation process. Spanish, a language I had heard all my life growing up in Spanish Harlem, was not coming easily to me. I had hoped to study it during the summer in preparation. If I could not master the language, what could I offer to those whom I was to serve? Further discouragement came in the many delays that seemed to prevent my translation of our skit on the "prodigal son" in time. It seemed that each person I had hoped to have translate the words into Spanish had a significant and understandable reason for not being able to accomplish this. If I could not do this for our team, I would be left with feelings of personal failure. These worries were so acute that they plagued me on a daily basis. I became doubtful and obsessive about so many things, including such trivia as which shoes to pack so that I would not stub my toes traveling the foreign landscape. All this was the work of Satan. For if you knew me as I think I know myself, these doubts are uncharacteristic of my spiritual perspective on life, my cognitive understanding of scriptural promises, and my usual personality. Because of these mental trials, the Lord taught me further lessons regarding His faithfulness and the armor of God against such attacks. Each time I meditated on the "helmet of salvation" as protection against my troubling thoughts, I felt a sudden calm. God also taught me the need for the indwelling of the Holy Spirit and to implement the fruits that are available. He taught me to understand the fruits of peace, patience, and kindness in a deeper way. Peace in the midst of turmoil, patience in the midst of provocation, and kindness during times of understandable anger were the three fruitful lessons I learned in preparation for Mexico.

Three New Reasons for Having Gone

María Isabel, a soft-spoken eight-year-old girl, revealed to Max, our missionary host, and myself that her uncle was an "hermano," a brother. In other words, he was a Christian. I had not seen this sweet girl who sat patiently to my left as numerous boisterous Mexican boys clamored around me begging for a free copy of St. John's gospel. It was not until Max pointed out to me that a young girl was quietly sitting next to me that I turned my attention to her. Her heart was so opened to the Lord that within the time of a brief conversation and the presentation of the gospel of Christ, María Isabel professed her faith. I wondered how God makes some things so easy while other issues in my life seem so overwhelming. In the grand scheme of things, the eternal life of an eight-year-old Mexican girl is worth infinitely more than anything I could obsess about.

Josefina and Alejandro, a young couple with one daughter, traveled all the way from Veracruz to work in the tomato fields at the Maracelis camp in San Vicente, Baja California. They told me they liked working at the camp. In their eyes, it was a steady, reliable form of employment. They attended a Catholic church in their hometown and seemed to have a genuine albeit reserved faith in the Lord. Their young daughter was suffering from "la gripe"—a cold—as well as stomach pains and vomiting. We led them to Dr. Fee, who was administering medical care that day, and the little girl received her treatment. About twenty minutes later, the grateful couple presented me with a large bag of tomatoes that they had harvested from the field. This brought tears to my eyes and a stabbing pain in my heart. How could I, who have the comforts of life far more than Alejandro and Josefina had ever known, deserve this act of generosity? It is an example of God's revelation to me that my cup runneth over. With an astonished "Gracias!" ("Thank you!"), I received the gift. The savory sweet taste of those tomatoes was unparalleled by any that I have eaten at home.

A sixty-three-year-old Mexican man, standing near me lamented, "No puedo comer" ("I cannot eat"). As a psychiatrist, it did not take long to evaluate his situation and diagnose clinical depression. To do this evaluation in another language, addressing another culture, was a professionally rewarding experience. I wrote down the names of the medicines that would help his situation, and he indicated that the next time he went to work in Los Angeles, he would try to obtain them. Never in the United States had I ever seen a patient so willing to wait a long time to fill a prescription. In an impoverished environment, this man was grateful to wait, knowing he had something to wait for that would help his condition. Many of his people wait a lifetime without getting the medical care they need. I was not able to give him the medicine he needed that day, but I did offer him spiritual medicine. Using the gospel of John booklet, I presented John 3:16. I explained to him that although his depressive illness caused him to see life and the future in a negative, pessimistic way, the Bible demonstrates very clearly that he is special and loved by God. Indeed, he is so loved that God sacrificed His only Son for him. He has the promise of the wonderful future of "la vida eterna" (eternal life). Without hesitation, he prayed the prayer of faith with Rudy, the Mexican missionary, and myself.

So if you ask me why I went to Mexico, I can give you three reasons: this depressed man, María Isabel, and the young couple from Veracruz. Furthermore, I could also give three reasons which include my personal growth in the three fruits of the Spirit: peace, patience, and kindness. Yet in my mind the most compelling reason for going on this Mexican mission trip was the conviction that God called me to go on that Sunday morning in the parking lot of the church. Because of this conviction, I have no regrets about making the trip.

Chapter 10

To Thailand and Beyond

But He said to me, "My grace is sufficient for you, for My power is made perfect in weakness." Therefore I [Paul] will boast all the more gladly in my weaknesses, so that Christ's power may rest on me. That is why, for Christ's sake, I delight in weaknesses, in insults, in hardships, in persecutions, in difficulties, for when I am weak, then I am strong.[1]

God has "stretched and used me" beyond my own imagination and I have grown in the process. Previously, I had been on short-term missions trips, where generally as a blind psychiatrist I had felt useful about 25 to 30 percent of the time. In Thailand, it was 98 percent. It is because missionary care (or "member care") has been proven to be God's calling for me, and I am happy for it.

Teaching is a joy and one of God's spiritual gifts. I wound up lecturing double the amount I expected, as I was being taken to various Thai Christian groups in town (Grace Thai Church, Harvest Dynamics Institute). Impromptu testimonies also took place over dinner and meetings with local co-workers in town. I met with Christians from McGilvery Theological Seminary (Payap University), others from Trinity International University (Deerfield, Illinois), Overseas Missionary Fellowship, and still others from the Christian Missionary Alliance who were serving in Chiang Mai. I also had the opportunity to worship at the International Church, a large expatriate English-speaking congregation which met in an open-air building that resounded with contemporary Christian music much like that from home. My travels did not end there, as I stopped in Kona, Hawaii, for medical meetings and Los Angeles, California, before returning to New York. In Los

Angeles, I also had the privilege of lecturing to over 100 Chinese pastors and their wives from the community at Logos Evangelical Seminary. I was blessed by their positive response and invitation of future speaking engagements in Taiwan and the United States.

Back to Chiang Mai—you can imagine my sense of being overwhelmed when I arrived alone at the conference center in the middle of 300 strangers attending the Christian Medical and Dental Association's (CMDA) commission. At first, I had to trust God that they were all Christian, missionaries, friendly, and wanting to share fellowship with me, but on the other hand they probably did not know how to deal with a blind person. But the appearance of 150 people at my first lecture ("Medical Update on Anxiety Disorders") instead of the anticipated 30, showed me that they cared very much. In a separate youth program, the children and teens also asked terrific questions about my blindness and how they could learn more in order to understand me. The two other workshops I led on "Coping with Stress and Transitions" and "Managing Worry and Anxiety" contained an audience with large hearts to share and learn about one another as they sought to serve Christ in the mission field. The mutual burdens shared gave us all a sense of support and unburdening. God permitted me to counsel a dozen people individually as we strolled through the lovely gardens, which were sprinkled with gentle waterfalls and dotted with small teakwood buildings of the Suan Bua Resort. At first I felt overwhelmed, jet-lagged, and ill prepared to counsel, but I knew that was the deception of the "enemy." When I realized once I started that the listening ear and the compassionate heart was therapeutic and all that was needed, I was amazed. Their gratitude and emotional relief told me that God truly is the "great physician." I hope and trust that He used me to make a difference in their lives and to encourage them in the vital work that they are doing. I have kept a brief diary of the scripture that was used in each case. I have also kept a diary of the times that God performed His miracles on my trip so I can discover who was praying for me at the time in the United States. So far, I have discovered four instances.

Anna Lee and her children were praying for me when she read the news that the Bangkok temperature was 95 degrees. It was a good thing, because I arrived at my hotel room after midnight and did not know how to turn on the air-conditioning. I did not want to disturb the hotel staff but then changed by mind. When I went to dial the operator on what I thought was the phone, I hit a button and heard the *whoosh* of air-conditioning pouring into the room.

Esther Louie had the housewife Bible study pray for my stomach, as they knew I might, in my food-tasting adventures, get sick in a foreign country. Their prayers occurred shortly after I did the risky thing of eating durian from a street vendor in Chinatown. For those acquainted with durian, you *know* that God truly answered that prayer, as I did not get sick! Durian is a foul-smelling fruit that paradoxically tastes like ambrosia to those who have acquired the taste for it. I hear that this tropical fruit is considered by legend to be the feces of a venerated sage. There is a definite resemblance! It has an odor akin to sewage waste and is banned from many hotels and restaurants.

A young boy, Wesley Yee, faithfully prayed for my safety each night, and I am sure God honored his prayers, as I came back to New York during the anticipation of a terrible spring northeaster. It turned out to be less than expected. Cliff prayed for me when I was traveling from Thailand to Tokyo for a five-hour layover before my next flight to Hawaii. It's a good thing he did, because the plane made two horrible turbulent attempts at landing in severe wind-shear conditions that caused everybody to scream as the oxygen masks deployed from above. I also prayed to the Lord during the forty-five minutes that we circled in the air. I was ready to be with Him if He wanted, but I asked that he would please not make it painful. I felt the comfort of Jesus as an illusion covering my chest as if to say, "Everything will be OK; trust Me." We finally landed safely, and during the five hours of wandering around the airport, God blessed me again when a United Airlines representative told me they were going to upgrade my seat to business class. The large, comfortable recliner, royal service, and the four-course meal complete with champagne made for a blissful night's sleep. God truly answers prayers!

As a blind person, I consider myself to be a poor networker. Yet God does the intervening on my behalf to accomplish His will. Here is an example: He kept allowing me to meet "Belinda." I first heard her testimony at a "Women in Medicine" meeting, and then at the pool where I was counseling someone else. "Belinda" introduced me to her two adopted sons who had been left to die due to a congenital abnormality. She lovingly rescued them from death and had helped them through many surgeries and much therapy. God put her in my presence for a third time when "Ophelia" asked me for a ride to inner Chiang Mai since she had heard that a Thai local was bringing me to speak at a Thai church. When I turned around to ask the identity of the other woman with "Ophelia," it was "Belinda" again. It seemed strange that in a meeting of 300 people I was bumping into her so often. After a few minutes of conversation, she became very excited when she learned that I was going to Kona, Hawaii, after this CMDA conference. She very determinedly urged me—and even made arrangements by telephone for me—to see the chair of the Counseling and Health Care Department at the University of the Nations, where she had trained. It turns out that this Christian university for missions was very close to the Outrigger Waikoloa, where I was staying in Hawaii. That "divine appointment" with Donna Livingston did occur, and much to our mutual benefit. "Belinda" felt that my book *"Martha, Martha": How Christians Worry* would be an important addition to their department, and so did I! God is truly my agent.

My son was led to pray for me every hour on the hour when he could remember. It was during one of these hourly moments that I met Clarene and Leslie at the Kona International Airport, where I originally lost my luggage. I was sitting alone for quite some time, waiting for the plane and feeling somewhat lonely and alienated from the surrounding people. Just as I was about to be escorted through agricultural customs, an elderly woman sat next to me and grabbed my hand. She said that she had been watching me and wanted to tell me I was very brave. I thanked her and then we got into conversation. Clarene was a retired nurse who trained at Loyola in Chicago. She struck me as a very gutsy lady also traveling alone. When she learned about my book, she became excited. Simultaneously, Leslie, a nurse who had also attended the CMDA conference, appeared. She saw my book and could not believe the topic. She felt it was just what she and her church in Chicago needed. I never thought I would be selling books at Kona Airport, but God must have known that this was the time to disperse *Mar-*

tha to Chicago and also to San Antonio, where Clarene now lives. Clarene told me that God must have sent her to me.

To sum up what I learned, in Corinthians I discovered that God's strength is made perfect in weakness—and I certainly felt weak enough to be awed by His power. I emphasized this fact when I spoke at Frosty's missionary kids program. Later, when I met with the teen group, I talked about how I must "walk by faith and not by *sight*." Traveling alone on this trip taught me again the truth of this passage: to God be all the glory.

Chapter 11

Fleece Fights Fear

Then the Spirit of the LORD came upon Gideon, and he blew a trumpet, summoning the Abiezrites to follow him.

He sent messengers throughout Manasseh, calling them to arms, and also into Asher, Zebulun and Naphtali, so that they too went up to meet them.

Gideon said to God, "If you will save Israel by my hand as you have promised—look, I will place a wool fleece on the threshing floor. If there is dew only on the fleece and all the ground is dry, then I will know that you will save Israel by my hand, as you said."

And that is what happened. Gideon rose early the next day; he squeezed the fleece and wrung out the dew—a bowlful of water.

Then Gideon said to God, "Do not be angry with me. Let me make just one more request. Allow me one more test with the fleece. This time make the fleece dry and the ground covered with dew."

That night God did so. Only the fleece was dry; all the ground was covered with dew.[1]

I am not an impulsive person. I spend time, prayer, and energy deliberating many of life's decisions, especially the ones that concern ministry, family, and profession. I thank God that He has given me a role model such as Gideon to follow, especially his use of the fleece in Judges 6:34-40. The fleece method has encouraged me to go to Kenya with my son without fear.

Called by the Lord to serve him with the Christian Medical and Dental Association (CMDA; previously known as the Christian

Medical and Dental Society, CMDS) in February 2002 in Kenya, I had no hesitation in saying yes to the invitation and making plans for my trip. At the advice of a medical colleague earlier in the year to *not* come alone into Nairobi and then Limuru, I was overjoyed when Brian, my son, told me he planned to graduate early from college and would accompany me on this mission and missionary care trip. Then September 11 happened. Although I never connected this horrible event to any danger I might face in Kenya, Cliff, my husband, started to hint that President Bush did not think Americans should go overseas.

Actually, it was more than hinting, because he kept saying it to me. I thank God that he did not tell me *not* to go, for then I would have obeyed. Although I had no fear of going alone, as a mother I did not have the heart to endanger my son in any way. So I prayed to God that He would show me as clearly as he did with the fleece to Gideon about Kenya. He did, through continuous confirmations even up to the last minute. I am going to share and thank God for the first two fleeces. The wet fleece had one bowl of water squeezed out of a parched environment. That is good stuff. Speaking of good stuff, the night before a women's conference, I was stuffing envelopes in preparation, along with some ladies from a local church. One of them introduced herself to me as Lillian Wong Suhu. We were talking about food from a great restaurant, and she told me that her company provides it to her for lunch every day. I said, "Wow! What a great job perk! Who do you work for?" She answered: British Airways. I told her I thought that was quite a coincidence, as my son and I were flying BA to Kenya for a mission trip. To that she instantly replied, "Give me your flight numbers and I will arrange for you to be in first class." Wow! Champagne, all the food you can eat, big reclining seats you can really sleep on, and incredible service—this *is* good stuff. Thank you, Lord, for the first fleece sign. Brian was also really happy when I told him the story. The next day, I spoke at the conference and then rushed to Alliance Graduate School of Counseling to teach my class. It was open house at Alliance, and soon my classroom began filling up with a lot of strangers visiting. At break time, a line formed at my lectern. Although I assumed they were my students waiting to ask me questions, I realized I was wrong when a woman with a thick Korean accent asked me for my phone number. I generally do not like giving out this information, especially to strangers, and balked. She was very insistent, and I think she wanted a relative to talk to me. I finally gave in, partly because I knew I still had a line of people waiting. I told her my number and immediately a voice behind her said, "I know that number!" What was going on here? She identified herself as a former patient of mine who was thinking of applying to the master's program in counseling. I rejoiced because this patient had worked so well in her therapy. I have often thought about and prayed for her since we finished. This was a clear sign that she was doing well, and she confirmed it. Immediately, the voice of the third person in line, a student of mine who happens to be from Nairobi, Kenya, indicated she was blessed to observe firsthand that what I had been teaching in my class really worked. Her deep feeling moved my heart as well, and I asked her if she would help me prepare for my trip to Kenya. She replied with an offer of all the help she could give, including teaching me the language Kiswahili! Praise the Lord! And jambo.[2] When I told Cliff about this in the car ride home, he was moved to tears. He finally felt at peace because He now knew that God wanted Brian and me to go to Kenya and that He would pave the way. Thank you, Lord, for the second fleece, dry as a bone in the wet environment of my husband's tears.

January 2002 was the month before I left for Kenya. Many details needed attention, including lecture preparation; ordering of materials; scheduling activities in Nairobi, London, and Limuru; packing; and the necessary prayer meetings for the trip. In the midst of this, I was asked to take on the presidency of Boro Pregnancy Counseling Center (BPCC) as this and another board position was being vacated. Such an important decision requires discernment of God's will and should not be undertaken just because it seems to be a good idea. Could I use Gideon's fleece method again? I did not want to overuse this technique or even use it out of biblical context. Yet when important decisions must be made in a short amount of time, what could I do? I asked the Lord to provide other board applicants, one Korean speaking and one Spanish speaking, to address important areas in our ministry. If He should so provide, I would consider it confirmation. My goal was not to give God an ultimatum but simply to discern by faith His will and to acknowledge His teaching in James that if any man lacks wisdom, he should go to God, who will provide it liberally. The Korean applicant came very quickly in the person of Lisha Sakhrani who felt called by the Lord to such a ministry. Praise God. However, weeks had lapsed from when I first asked God for the demonstration of His fleece in October 2001. Finally, on New Year's Eve, I received a message on my answering machine from Soraya Cina telling me that after months of prayer she felt called by God to leave her comfort zone and join the BPCC board. Praise the Lord for this Venezuelan, Spanish-speaking symbol of Gideon's fleece in the BPCC ministry. Without hesitation, I informed the rest of the board that God had called me to accept the presidency.

Chapter 12

Africa: Why I Go, Why I Cry

Weep with those who weep.[1]

Missionary care, defined as that branch of ministry that encompasses the care of the psychological, spiritual, and physical health of Christians on the mission field, is an important focus of today's Christian doctor. Physicians such as psychiatrists Dr. Jarrett Richardson, Dr. Barney M. Davis Jr., and the late Dr. David L. Stewart have contributed greatly to the development of this field as they serve and have served the needs of missionaries. Missionary care may include help in adjustment to their surroundings, marital issues, family life, transitions, illnesses, and, most important, their spiritual needs. One organization, the Christian Medical and Dental Association, attends to the specific needs of medical missionaries through its Commission of Continuing Medical and Dental Education (CMDE). This project, which began twenty-three years ago, has provided for the Continuing Medical Education (CME) accreditation for the medical missionaries in Africa, Asia, and throughout the world. This is done in conjunction with providing biblical feeding through inspiring preachers, Christian counseling, and a program of fellowship and support to the spouses and children. Alternating between Asia and Africa, the highly qualified members from the United States bring up-to-date medical information to full-time missionaries, with some faculty enthusiastically returning on a yearly basis.

Dr. Marvin Jewell, a pioneer and visionary in this ministry since its inception, has worked faithfully in this endeavor.

In 1976, Dr. Jewell, president of CMS [Christian Medical Society], appointed David (Stewart) to chair the Missions Committee. Their focus on the needs of missionary members culminated in establishing these CMDS-CMDE Conferences with the first one convening in Monrovia, Liberia, January 1978 with a faculty of 13 and student body of 65.[2]

Since then, there has been an annual CMDA-CMDE meeting for the past twenty-three years. Mary Jane, Dr. Jewell's wife and the administrative secretary for the conferences, has this to say: "We are here to serve the missionaries for the vital work that they do." This work is so gratifying for them that Dr. Jewell concluded at the outbreak of the Gulf War, when he was preparing to leave for the CMDE, that this ministry was "worth dying for." The conferees find enormous encouragement, fellowship, and camaraderie while getting their CME credits without having to interrupt their work by going stateside. Their gratitude and glowing evaluations have blessed the faculty and organizers with a zeal to continue the work. A practical question to ask doctors is why do they go every year to serve in the CMDE commission? Dr. Martha Housholder, a dermatologist who teaches and has served almost every year since 1984, states, "There is no other setting where I can be exposed to the richness of Christian fellowship, music, and medicine . . . this is a unique blend in Christian ministry." Many others echo the same sentiment as the basis for their service to the Lord's missionaries. Yet there is a better question than "What makes doctors go?" It is this: "What makes us cry?"

As a physician, I have trained myself not to cry easily. So it is only when a situation touches me in some inner way that is so profoundly sad or utterly joyful and often deeply spiritual that my tears begin to flow. Last year, when I was invited to serve the missionaries in Thailand by teaching the update on anxiety disorders, teaching workshops on transitions and managing worry, and partnering with Dr. Jarrett Richardson on the counseling team, I cried a flood of tears. At the beautiful countryside of the Suan Bua Resort where the conference was held, I shed tears of empathy for the missionaries I heard from, tears of admiration for their perseverance despite hardship, tears of sadness for the plight of the Thai people ravaged by AIDS, and tears of thanksgiving for our sovereign God who gives strength for the task. The experience was so powerful for me that when I was invited again to Kenya this year, I knew without hesitation that the Lord had once again given me a privilege to serve Him in this unique way.

Recently, a memorable night of tears at the Brackenhurst Baptist International Conference Center occurred on Tuesday, February 19, 2002, when I heard about the life of Dr. Martha Stewart, missionary doctor for over thirty years in Nigeria. This petite, elderly woman of eighty-three years took the podium that night and recounted the many stories of incredible medical work in a mission hospital treating the medical needs and catastrophes seen commonly in Nigerian women but rarely encountered stateside. Her courage, perseverance, and tenacity in dealing with the daunting obstetrical and gynecological problems in a medically primitive setting did not seem possible in this sweet, gentle, southern lady. Yet her strength emanated that night as she spoke of her zeal for the Lord and commitment to spreading His message of love through healing. Perhaps the best description of Dr. Stewart's life was narrated by Dr. Jarrett Richardson, who introduced her and was acknowledged as her first and perhaps most important work in Nigeria—the attendance of his birth to Dr. Margaret Richardson, a fellow medical missionary. Here is what he had to say:

> Nigerian interns called Martha "the iron woman." She could outlast the young men who often gave up after ten or twelve hours, and she kept going up to fourteen hours, with only an occasional sip of water.
>
> Martha had a way of turning a social occasion into a spiritual occasion. When she was [the] Francis Jones [Guesthouse] hostess she usually had a plan for dinner parties. She would say something like, "Let's not talk about the weather or politics or what we don't like about someone—let's take a few minutes to think and then go around the table and tell about a time in the life of Jesus when you would especially wish to be with him."
>
> She had a way of making ordinary circumstances have a spiritual tone.

She cries easily over beauty, not so much for suffering or sorrow. A gesture, a musical phrase, a lovely sight would and still does bring tears. She still will be moved by the way verses are written in a new translation of the Bible, and call up a friend to share her joy.

Martha played organ at the Oke Ilerin (Hill of the Elephant Church) in Ogbomosho—and the people often would say, "such a small person—such a mighty music she makes."

She and my mother were good friends—both female physicians who had to earn respect in their work in Africa yet both of whom remained feminine in the best ways throughout their long and arduous careers. She and my mother both attended the first CMDS-CMDE in Liberia in 1978, and were colleagues in Ogbomosho for thirty years—caring for each other's families and Martha delivering my mother of me in 1947.

Martha began studying Greek at age eighty and at eighty-three is taking the second year again—she is able to read Romans in the original Greek now. Once recently when she was out of class for a few days with the flu, she returned to hear—"Dr. Stewart, when you were absent we voted you most likely to succeed."[3]

Dr. Martha then proceeded to share her thoughts about her late husband, Dr. David L. Stewart.

David Lawrence Stewart was born to missionary parents in Japan on December 10, 1924. Orphaned by the death of both parents by the time he was five years old, he and three older siblings were raised by an aunt who had been a missionary in China.

David was a graduate of Asbury College and the University of Louisville School of Medicine. After internship he and his wife Laura and their first child went to Burundi, Africa, to begin a new medical mission. Operating first out of tents, he established a thriving eighty-bed hospital. Early in David's service there was a hiatus that included surgical resection of his colon cancer in the U.S., plus two years of follow-up observation during which he completed a residency in psychiatry. They returned to pick up full responsibilities and he also delivered three of his four children, planted churches, brought in running water and electrical power, and was generally the sole physician at the Murore Hospital.

Leaving full-time mission work in 1961, David and Laura and their four children returned to Louisville, Kentucky, where he practiced psychiatry. Laura died in 1979 and in 1981 David married Martha.

Dr. Stewart directed the 1989 Malaysia Symposium and was preparing for the next one in Kenya for 1990 when he died in November of 1989, ending an earthly life that was so full and well lived and touching so many with blessing and healing. These are the memories that will go on inspiring others to do honor to our Lord.[4]

At the conclusion of Dr. Martha's lecture, there was a standing ovation for this inspiring woman and her late husband. There was not a dry eye in the audience of many physicians, public health workers, and missionaries who have served in equally difficult situations. The remarkable work of the Lord in this special woman served to strengthen each listener and infuse them with new conviction. I knew I would return to New York in a few days to my practice and teaching responsibilities, but the life of Dr. Martha Stewart and the tears I shed that night inspired by her story had a profound effect on the ministry and, yes, the mission I have in the urban field. Her testimony infused new life in how I will serve God here at home. Her story strengthened my commitment to the ministry I have of serving women in a crisis pregnancy center. Her account of her work in Nigeria will be a model for how God's work will be carried on in our ministry. Deeply touched by how the Lord used this woman, the tears shed that night must have reflected something in the inner core of every Christian physician in their desire to serve Christ in medicine.

Chapter 13

Blind Professor

"Think BIG," one of my students told her visually handicapped sister. "I've got this professor at the seminary, and you'd never know she's blind when she teaches. She travels all over the world and lectures. Sometimes I forget that she is blind." I keep scratching my head every time a student or someone in the audience tells me that they "forget" that I am blind. How can that be? I carry a cane with me to the podium. Sometimes I discuss my illness when I tell my life story as part of the presentation. How can they forget? But they do. I know it is true because many of them raise their hands to ask questions even though I warn them from the beginning that I cannot acknowledge them when they raise their hands. Instead, they are instructed, "Blurt out your questions when you have them. I do not mind interruptions, and I do not consider it rude in my lectures." Yet they forget, and countless observers tell me it happens a lot. Others sheepishly confess that they have done the up then down—"Oops!"—arm exercises in my class. A keen observer finally explained it to me. The scanning motion of my eyes when talking to individuals may be disconcerting, as I am trying to locate the voice and try to make a reasonable facsimile of eye-to-eye contact. But this scanning is suddenly transformed to a vision of "comfort in the place of presentation" because the motion of my eyes works well in an audience situation, giving the illusion that each individual is being spoken to personally. Of course, the content of my rehearsed, studied, and memorized lecture needs to be interesting and well delivered, and for the most part I have enjoyed good success in this area. So as my students tell me that they forget I am blind, I now understand their perspective.

There are some humorous stories from them as well. For example, my first class of students was thankful and yet confused about how I knew it was time to give them a break or end class. They saw me look at the back of the classroom where the clock was and then dismiss them. What they did not know was simultaneous to "glancing" at the back wall, I made a sweeping motion with my left hand and pressed a button on my "talking watch," which then whispers the time in my left ear. This motion is so automatic with me that to others it may appear as if I am smoothing back my hair and not trying to hear the time. Some of the students find the following funny, and others are appalled. In order to take attendance, I ask them all to remain in the same seats for the entire semester, such as what is done in law schools. At each class, they are requested to tell me their names at the beginning, which is comparable to a roll call. I make a mental note of the absent, but I remind them that if they do come in late to let me know upon arrival. Some of the students take this very seriously and admonish the ones that stray from their assigned seats. As for latecomers, a few of them never let me know. Some have suggested that they "sneak in and act as if they were there from the beginning." I tend to believe many are simply uncomfortable interrupting a lecture in progress, especially if they are late. Whatever the reason, it is often a focus of student comment. To reassure them, I tell them it is quite simple, almost mathematical, but I can tell who is late by subtracting the list present in the beginning from the final mental list of students I make as new additional voices are heard during the class. Thank God I have pretty good voice recognition skills. My class is generally interactive and emphasizes student participation. These conditions make it very difficult to fool me, although I suspect if someone really wanted to do it, he or she could devise a way. What good would it do? It would only be to their detriment in their studies.

Another comical misperception is revealed in the following e-mail from a student:

Dr. Eng,

One funny thing that stands out for me regarding you as my teacher occurred several times. Every so often, in class you would appear to be reading from a document. Myself and my fellow classmates would sit there looking quite perplexed. How can you be blind and read from a document? Was this a special kind of blindness? I'm not sure if you explained this phenomenon to us or not but most of us were thrown off for much of the semester! I later learned the truth about this at a chapel service where I got a look at what you were 'reading' from . . . it was basically a blank sheet of paper! I guess the joke was on us.

With love, Chantelle

Teaching the seminary and graduate students provides me with a forum to integrate issues of faith and psychology in a personally meaningful way. Also gratifying is my work instructing the medical students on the psychosocial aspects of obstetrics and gynecology which addresses the interface of the two specialties important to the needs of women. As assistant professor of psychiatry in the Department of Obstetrics and Gynecology at Cornell-Weill Medical College, I have delivered lectures to numerous groups of students who are learning about the treatment of women in the hospital. It is important for them to learn about the emotional needs of these women as well as their physical needs. I sometimes wonder how the Cornell students feel encountering a blind physician as their teacher, but I have never asked. I think we in medicine tend to address the task at hand and often there is very little time or room for such personal questions. I did, however, obtain feedback from Dr. Robert Post, the past chairman of obstetrics and gynecology at New York Hospital Queens Medical Center where I teach. He says, "The students always expressed positive responses to your meetings. They also expressed admiration for your overcoming the disability and your positive approach to everything."[1]

Let me highlight one of my most special experiences as a blind teacher. I had the privilege to advise and then teach a student who shared a similar visual handicap. As soon as I met her, I sensed God had brought her into my life for a good purpose and I wanted to be used by Him for it. She explained her struggles as a student trying to master a body of clinical information, which, as it turns out, she was good at because of her conscientiousness. However, the increased difficulties in applying that knowledge to the clinical situation in internship was daunting to her. It seemed to me that the main problem was the logistics of not seeing well in clinical and group situations where the sighted have an advantage by being able to connect easily with patients or other staff. The visually handicapped need to make extra effort and take more time to do this simple task. Because these small but seemingly insurmountable factors, which have nothing to do with being a competent counselor, interfere, their discouraging effect can generalize to a feeling of inadequacy in all areas. I was exposed to the same issues in my early professional training, and I confronted them with the mantra, "I may be blind, but I am not stupid. God has put me here for a purpose, and I will be teachable. I am willing to work hard, but no amount of travail or mental fortitude is going to make me see." I gently informed the institution that I would try to help them help me by being their educator as to how to help the blind learn. The psychiatry department's receptivity to this plan made for a mutually beneficial learning experience for us all, culminating with my graduation from the program. The concept of leveling the playing field was very much needed to accomplish this, and it was very much needed in my student's training. I conveyed this idea to the program director, but how could I get the student to trust this as true and not to personalize her difficulties? It required much more than simply communicating this information; it required modeling on my part. I had the opportunity to do so when she enrolled in my class the following semester.

The awesome changes began at first subtly then quite apparently as if through a divine transformation. One of the other students remarked, "I don't know what happened. Something changed. I got closer to her. It was as if she were a real person." Of course, this student was always a "real person," but the perceptions of others may have been distorted by her reticence. These perceptions may also reflect society's ignorance of the presence and contribution of the disabled. Anyway, God used my disability for the good of us both, and it worked miracles for her self-image. She says it best in the following e-mail:

Dear Dr. Eng:

I was reminded of two verses. The first passage I am reminded of is in St. Paul's letter to the Corinthians where Paul
tells us that he pleaded to the Lord three times to heal him. He
records that the Lord says "My grace is sufficient for you, for My
power (strength) is made perfect in weakness." Paul continues
to write, "Therefore, most gladly I will rather boast in my infirmi-
ties that the power of Christ may rest upon me." The second, in
St. Paul's letter to Colossians, he writes, "And whatever you do,
do it heartily, as to the Lord and not to men, knowing that from
the Lord you will receive the reward of the inheritance, for you
serve the Lord Christ."

Dr. Eng, I really saw God's power in your weakness. I was always amazed, despite your inability to see, the material was presented with excellence. It was clear, organized and expressed
perfectly. I always thought to myself, how could Dr. Eng present
so brilliantly without any notes or outline (overheads) like the
other professors? I learned a great deal through your example
both personally and professionally. After meeting with you and
being in your course, I felt hopeful and encouraged. I saw how
you counseled (modeled counseling in our class) and lectured
with excellence. I knew that I wanted and needed to strive for
that and needed not to use my disability as an excuse. You
showed me that a disability (though it has physical limitations)
could be strength. I learned throughout the past year not to be
ashamed but to communicate honestly and directly about my
limitations and God's strength was vividly seen in my interac-
tions.

My internship supervisor commented, "How rewarding it is to
have seen [me] change, to become a woman of confidence and
poise." Thanks, Dr. Eng—for your example."

This touching letter brought tears to my eyes as it represents my
most deeply satisfying legacy in my role of blind professor.

Although I teach courses on anxiety and mood disorders and
issues in counseling women, the satisfaction of having the students learn this material is greatly enhanced by the other lessons
they learn. My blindness has caused some of the more reflective
students to realize how much they inadvertently judge and stereo-

type others on the basis of appearances. First impressions are so natural and immediate for the sighted that it takes time before these impressions are corroborated, modified, or completely reversed by reality. Sometimes there is no opportunity for these impressions to be validated or altered; the judgment is pronounced "etched in memory's stone." A student wondered how I "imaged" the individual class members in my mind. She concluded that I could not rush to a conclusion as she tended to by appearances alone, and therefore I must pause to listen to the person's heart and keenly focus on the content of his or her expressed thoughts. She observed that my powers of listening were infinitely more keen and thorough than were hers and those of the sighted world. After all, the sighted can afford to, and often do, pay less or partial attention to what is being said because they have the recourse to read the notes later or to see the visual clues at another time. Blind listeners do not have that luxury and are often more attentive to the sounds of their surroundings and what people say. This is indeed true for me and for a number of the blind, well-functioning people I know.

Psychological and spiritual lessons learned in the company of a blind professor are so surprising to me and remind me of the constant flow of wisdom given by God. This excerpt from a student's letter will demonstrate this.

Hi Dr. Eng:

What a gift you gave us all! Studying under a blind professor offered me the marvelous challenge of revisiting and exploring some issues in my own soul. As I mentioned, I grew up in Africa, the daughter of wonderful parents whom I rarely saw—basically I felt myself to be "orphaned" as many others of that time were as missionary kids. Living my childhood in chronic grief due to separation has taken its toll. There have been times in my life when it has been difficult to connect the love of God my Father with the idea of my parents serving Him overseas and thus denying me of much needed parental care in my childhood. Meeting up with a person like you serves me with a wonderful challenge of yet again rummaging through my own life and attitudes and asking myself those tough questions about my attitude toward pain and suffering. I have experienced both holding on to pain and becoming angry and bitter, and other times letting go of my need to know the "why" and simply choosing to forgive, accept, and place my trust in my heavenly Father. You gave us a shining example of the latter . . .

With gratefulness for having had my life enriched because of your blindness and the way you have chosen to live with it and accept it and allow God to shape and mold you in His image, I remain, your friend,

Lois Shellrude

Since I became blind, I have felt that God indeed has made me "special" in a positive sense—not that I am any more special than anyone else, but special nonetheless. It consists of the uniqueness found in all His children as outlined in the Bible. It also is anchored in the combined love and support of many friends, family, students, and even strangers I have met. They all have added to my strong sense of worth and value at being used as His instrument. This kind of support can mislead one into a false sense of pride as it tickles one's narcissism. But I am acutely aware that pride goes before the fall and arrogance is the one thing that will lead to a loss of my vast supply of supportive people in my life. So warned about that trap, let me beg the reader's forgiveness and indulge in recording one more contribution from a student.

Reflections of a Student of a Blind Teacher
by Diane Sardanopoli

I remember the first day that I met Dr. Elaine Eng on August 26, 2000, at the Alliance Graduate School of Counseling orientation. She introduced herself to the counseling students and shared with them her experience of losing her sight. I remember that I was in awe as I listened to her speak. I saw the joy and humility that filled her as she spoke gently but firmly to those of us who would embark on a life-changing journey to serve Christ and counsel His hurting and broken people. I remember thinking to myself what a testimony she is to the love and glory of God. I realized that Dr. Eng is a woman who has an intimate relationship with her Savior and that she has come to truly rely on God for her life and placed her trials, obstacles, and all her experiences in the Lord's sovereign hands.

I was amazed that (in my opinion) for a woman that had a very difficult trial to bear, Dr. Eng was truly praising God and thanking Him for her life. One of the points that she had discussed was that in some way she saw her blindness as a blessing. She had talked about the fact that when she began to lose her sight she needed to stay home. She had said that if it wasn't for her losing her sight, she probably would not have gotten time to stay home with her children when they were still very young. That statement really encouraged me. Even though I imagined that she must have struggled deeply with losing her sight and perhaps was at first angry about the situation, I believed that she had committed her situation to the Lord. Even in the midst of her trial, the Lord opened her spiritual eyes and allowed her to see the blessing in a difficult situation.

When I saw Dr. Eng that day and heard her speak, I thought to myself, *I hope that I have the opportunity to be taught by this godly woman.* I believe that God allowed me that day to see the courage, strength, love, and humility that He has given Dr. Eng in great abundance. Her talk really inspired me and confirmed to me that no matter what obstacles or trials God allows in our lives, He will never leave us. The Lord will give us the strength and the grace to persevere and receive victory in our life if we will humble ourselves and turn to Him. Another wonderful gift that I observed in Dr. Eng that day was the wisdom and intelligence that the Lord has given her. Among the many words of encouragement and wisdom that she imparted to us, there were a few in particular that really touched me. Dr. Eng had said, "God is not so concerned with your ability as He is with your availability. Allow Him to work in your life and in you and express Himself through you. Abandon yourself to God saying, God, Here I am!" I believe this statement is both true and spoken from the wisdom and revelation that God had given her through her own life experiences. Also, observing Dr. Eng that day, I could see that she genuinely cared about the students and their individual relationships with the Lord. As I went through school and counseled at a psychiatric hospital for a year, Dr. Eng's words became a reality in my life. I strongly believe that God wants our hearts, our hopes, and our failures. He wants us to give Him everything and to be open and willing to do His will in our lives and in the lives of others. I have experienced in my own life that if I allow God into my life and my circumstances, He will bless me beyond what I can imagine or think. He has used me in others' lives. He has healed me emotionally from hurt and suffering that I have endured. He has changed me and is still in the process of changing me into the woman of God that He has planned for me to become.

I was excited when I had the opportunity to take Dr. Eng's Anxiety and Mood Disorders class at the Alliance Graduate School of Counseling (AGSC). While in the classroom, I was able to see on a daily basis the love, kindness, and compassion that the Lord has poured into her. The same joyful and courageous spirit that I saw when she spoke at the AGSC orientation was very visible in her classroom. In class, as she spoke about the Lord and the Word of God, I could sense and hear in her voice the genuine love that she has for Jesus. Her praises and joy to the Lord motivated me and inspired me in both my professional and personal life. I also observed and admired the humility and gentleness that she demonstrated to her students on a daily basis. I also realized that along with these blessed qualities the Lord has also given her the ability to speak firmly with wisdom and confidence in Him.

I was humbled as I sat in Dr. Eng's classroom and watched her teach. I realized that no matter what experiences we go through in life, we need to have a grateful heart and be thankful to God and speak and sing our praises to Him and live our lives with a joyful and loving spirit. Dr. Eng's life and ministry as a counselor is a testimony to this truth.

Another wonderful quality that I experienced as her student was her willingness to always go the extra mile and help her students in answering questions and encouraging them to excel in their endeavor to be a Christian Counselor. In particular, I remember when Dr. Eng encouraged and affirmed my writing ability and suggested that I send a copy of one of my essays to the American Association of Christian Counselors for publication. I really appreciated the prayers, time, and energy that she put into helping me with the essay. That experience allowed me to see even more clearly the loving, encouraging, and joyful spirit that the Lord has given her. Dr. Eng has been a wonderful blessing in my life and I thank God for her.

Chapter 14

World Trade Center Tragedy: From Helplessness to Healing

> Then Job replied: "Even today my complaint is bitter; his
> hand is heavy in spite of my groaning.[1]

Post-traumatic stress disorder is triggered by a life-threatening situation that results in intense fear and a sense of helplessness. The events of September 11, 2001, fulfill this definition in dimensions previously unknown to our profession. Countless individuals barely escaped with their lives in the World Trade Center (WTC) attack, only to be rendered helpless and further traumatized by the loss of thousands of colleagues and rescue workers. Billions around the world were left shocked and horrified as they were inundated with scenes of burning towers and people leaping out of windows for a momentary respite from their fiery agony. The television cameras replayed the trauma over and over again, producing in many a sense of helpless agitation and others a heroic, indescribable need to do something, anything to address the human suffering and their own personal identification with the extraordinary pain. Can there be any relief in this cataclysmic tragedy? In the early days following the attack, many people flocked to help in some way. Some were turned away politely or asked to wait because there was already too much offered or there was not enough infrastructure to collect the blood or other donations. Many did not know how they could help and arrived on the scene with what they had, a desire to offer their help in the midst of profound helplessness. Others struggled to make sense of this tragedy for themselves while victims and their families found no sense in it at all. As doctors prepared to heal those that could be saved, some of their colleagues waited for patients that never arrived. "We discharged a lot of people . . . in order to provide beds for the expected injured and set up all sorts of extra staffing for psychiatric emergencies, but nobody came," said Dr. Carol Bernstein. Only about 100 patients from the disaster were treated at Bellevue that morning, a telling sign of the later massive loss of life.[2] If any event were to create a sense of helplessness in the nation's psyche, the WTC tragedy was the penultimate. It seemed to deal a blow to our Christian beliefs, bloodying our souls as well as the rubble of the fallen buildings. Chinua Achebe in his book, *No Longer at Ease,* states, "Real tragedy is never resolved. It goes on hopelessly forever."[3] What can the time period following September 11 reveal about his statement?

I remember our church's angst in finding the missing. Frantic phone calls permitted us to find some of our loved ones and friends who made it but left a list of the missing whom we hunted for and obsessed about for weeks. Long lines formed at information centers, around hospitals, the armory, and other stations. Words of comfort suggested that they are somewhere, probably in an emergency room or at the Liberty Park makeshift station, and just have not been entered into a database yet. Soon these words rang hollow as the building rubble burned and very few survivors were found. Even Christian quotes felt at times to be hollow platitudes as a mother and father cried for their missing son. So many prayers were uttered looking for the missing, for God, and for His answers during this dark and informationless time. It is reminiscent of Job's lament: "But if I go to the east, he is not there; if I go to the west, I do not find him. When he is at work in the north, I do not see him; when he turns to the south, I catch no glimpse of him."[4]

My own personal experiences were no different from many. Shaken by a friend's desperate search for a missing daughter from the 96th floor, I was mobilized in an effort to reach every contact in the hospitals I knew, and I sought to comfort the family—and probably myself—by saying that God knows where she is and she will be found. But the chilling realization came slowly: while God did know where she was, we will not be able to find her on this earth. What unspeakable helplessness is this challenge to faith. In the course of looking for the missing, I made a new friend. We were physicians who were to have our first meeting together that day of September 11 to discuss how we could collaborate in working on health education in our community. The voice mail came in one hour before our meeting time: "Dr. Eng, I am sorry, I have to cancel. My son was in the World Trade Building and I cannot reach him." My maternal heart was sickened, but my physician side energized me to help this stranger-made-friend-by-circumstance. Over the next two weeks, we labored together to search the city for our missing loved ones, each trying to find encouragement for our own and each other's family, to no avail. I remarked to her by phone, as we had never met face to face despite our many phone conversations, that "with God nothing is impossible." She held onto that comment even to the day of her son's memorial. Christian platitude or encouraging words—it is so difficult to discern.

Many physicians are drawn to the idea of rescuing others predominantly through medicine but also through any other means. We as a group have been motivated to make tremendous sacrifices of time and leisure to devote ourselves to rescuing, healing, and eliminating suffering. We do not do well with helplessness or the unsolvable crises of life. For the Christian and non-Christian doctor, the World Trade Center disaster posed a challenge to our rescue fantasies which drives us to bandage, medicate, and suture the wounded that would flow freely to our sanctuaries of healing. Yet what happens when the supply of patients is so disproportionately miniscule compared to the numbers of dead bodies and body parts carried out by the fatigued rescue workers and firefighters? Even more incomprehensibly disproportionate were the numbers of people remaining in the ashes of the burning rubble. It leaves physicians challenged with a troubling helplessness, much like my first experience of losing a patient to an illness that was incurable. I will also never forget my profound sadness when Mrs. M. suddenly died before me, postop. The tears betrayed my vulnerable interior as a young resident. We as physicians all have such despairingly helpless moments in our training that never go away but are wounds that become more calloused with repeated exposure to death—wounds that may have even started in an early life encounter with sickness and death that propelled the entry into the medical career. Medicine for some may have been an attempt to emotionally master the helplessness due to childhood experiences of sickness or dying. Death is the enemy that recapitulates childhood fears and trauma.

As a blind physician, I have often viewed my handicap as a challenge to be overcome. For the purposes of my WTC reflections, it has become a paradigm for helplessness. My immediate response to the horrendous attack was to prepare myself for the battle through the means of healing, but what could I do? I was no longer able to do surgery, no longer even able to see wounds that needed bandaging. I was barely able to see the family member that needed comfort. How could I help? I had to wrestle with my insurmountable limitations before I could even lift a finger to help. I found this at times intolerable, producing a needless, self-condemnation of powerful but of unclear origins. I, like Job, asked, "Would he oppose me with great power? No, he would not press charges against me. There an upright man could present his case before him, and I would be delivered forever from my judge."[5]

Were I not able to utilize God's medicinal tool of intercessory prayer and the modern devices of the telephone and e-mail, through which the balm of comforting words, a listening ear, and the prescriptive of helpful advice could be made, my helplessness would be overwhelming. My blindness became the paradigm to understand the helpless reactions of many individuals to the WTC crisis. So many rescuers could not see the bodies trapped by the rubble. So many family members could and will never see their loved ones. So many doctors did not see the survivors they anticipated. So many people could not see how to make sense of any of this. Our country never saw the approach of the enemy until it was too late. Christians grappled to obtain God's vision in order to make sense of this tragedy. Non-Christians sought insight through their yet undiscovered spiritual selves. If not, they needed to see the face of the terrorists, the initially unknown and unseen villains who perpetrated this crime. As my blindness gives way to insight, so did our nation's collective myopia cause it to put on the corrective glasses of leadership, humanitarianism, perseverance, and faith during this tragedy. We are still in that process, with more to be revealed. Like Job, we yearn for clarity: "If only I knew where to find him; if only I could go to his dwelling! I would state my case before him and fill my mouth with arguments. I would find out what he would answer me, and consider what he would say."[6]

My professional career as a psychiatrist was a double-edged sword—or perhaps "scalpel" would be the better term. Although it was the instrument through which I would perform therapeutic acts for those whose lives were traumatized by the September 11 disaster, it was also the setting through which I would be repeatedly traumatized in my own psyche. "Nothing in my life so far has prepared me to face the sights, sounds, smells and emotions that accompanied the horror of Sept. 11," said Spencer Eth, MD, who is the vice chair of the Department of Psychiatry at St. Vincent's Hospital.[7] This hospital was one of the closest to the disaster and took care of many of the injured.

The effects of repeated trauma are seen in the person glued to the news, repeatedly visualizing the attack with all its horrors and wondering why he or she cannot sleep at night when the images and his or her own anxiety keep him or her up. I, too, felt that there was no escape from the repeated exposures to patients' anxieties, grief, and their existential despair. I have cried many tears since 9/11, but I do not know how many were my own and how many were for others. Could they really be separated in such a national phenomenon? My professional career was a tool, but it was also a burden just like the dilemma faced by all those steadfast, tireless volunteers who served at ground zero. They were burdened by the misery but would never have chosen any option other than to be there and help. It also reflects the conflicts of those determined firefighters, vigilant about digging their brothers and sisters out of the rubble but deeply wounded by the constant exposure to the reality of death on a massive scale. How much helplessness can people bear in trying to help?

A pivotal point of God's healing process in me occurred at the Trauma Response and Grief Training Conference sponsored in part by the American Association of Christian Counselors. This was held at Calvary Baptist Church in New York City on October 23 and 24, 2001. Standing in the emotional rubble of hurting New York church leaders, pastors, teachers, and clinicians, I joined a long list of speakers to minister to the 1,100 attendees in a program of education, ministry, fellowship, prayer, counseling, and resource distribution to the faith community of New York. I spoke on the topic, "Recognizing Anxiety Disorders in the Aftermath of the World Trade Center Disaster," joining with others who spoke on their areas of expertise. Dwight Bain, Tim Clinton, Larry Crabb, Archibald Hart, David Epstein, Ron Hawkins, Ed Hindson, June Hunt, Diane Langberg, H. B. London, Michael Lyles, Gordon MacDonald, Josh McDowell, Beth Moore, George Ohlschlager, Les Parrott, Molly Shotzberger, Gary Smalley, E. Glenn Wagner, and H. Norman Wright were just some of the "spiritual rescue workers" I had the privilege to serve with in this faith-based project. The experience, replete with tears, compassion, suffering, rejoicing, despair, and hope, was memorable and transforming not only for the audience but also for the speakers and the many volunteers who worked tirelessly to put this conference together in just three weeks. For me, it provided a vehicle for helping in a Christian context and thus began my process of healing, as the Lord was clearly presiding over the room. He was the great physician over the surgical arena of His people's wounded souls. There the healer met the other healers who needed to be helped while helping the helpless. His words were spoken that made sense out of a senseless massacre, a tragedy which at first glance could not make sense in a Christian nation. Yet He reminded us of His own trauma, the tortured death of His own Son to procure our salvation and spiritual healing. His higher perspective illuminated the surgical field and the Word became the instrument promising a better prognosis for the weakened souls. All this was integrated with the psychological tools that He has generously given His counselors to understand and employ. His wisdom, comfort, and love as shown through His followers were clearly demonstrated that day. It initiated my own therapy as "a wounded healer."

"God is back," declares Peggy Noonan. She writes: "In the wake of an atrocity, he shows he hasn't forsaken New York. God is back. He's bursting out all over. It's a beautiful thing to see. Random data to support the assertion: In the past 17 days, since the big terrible thing, our country has, unconsciously but quite clearly, chosen a new national anthem. It is 'God Bless America,' the song everyone sang in the days after the blasts to show they loved their country."[8] Not only do we have a new national anthem, we have had many opportunities to sing it. We have openly proclaimed the name of Christ and His word at the thousands of memorials and funerals for the dead.

Jennifer, a young Christian woman in her twenties, had already accomplished much service for the Lord when she was taken to be with Him on September 11. Although truly missed by her family, friends, and church members, her memorial service, just like her life, was a praiseful offering of dedication, worship, and commitment to the gospel of Jesus Christ. The attendees, soaked with the tears of loss and pain, were quickly bathed with the salve of hope from heaven, where Jennifer now resides. I left the service with a feeling of renewal and fearlessness that stared at the face of any terrorist or biological weapon that would dare to thwart my role in the work of the Lord. It was Jennifer's legacy that showed me the way. She had exemplified bravery, generosity, and faith in her mission mindedness. In my own preparation to serve with the Christian Medical and Dental Association's CME program in Kenya, February 2002, I was but momentarily paused by the news item, "Saudi exile Osama bin Ladin, who is charged with leading a decade-long worldwide conspiracy to kill Americans and destroy U.S. government property . . . Twenty-two men have been charged in the bombings of the embassies in Kenya and Tanzania."[9] Even though the embassy bombings took place in Kenya, Jennifer's memoriam quickly obliterated any doubt or fear about going. Let me share one of the poignant excerpts taken from her tributes:

. . . a wonderful sister, friend, mentor, and a woman of God, Jennifer, you will truly be missed. I know I'll never be able to find another person as beautiful as you—spiritually, physically, and mentally. You were spiritually strong. What role did you not take in church? Never did you say no to serving God. Bible studies, Sunday school, worship team, and even scraping the floor. Everything you did, you gave Him your best. Even helping me lead Bible study. You were there to guide me. You always took time and took the extra step to help. You were always there to encourage your brothers and sisters to do more for God. You were truly a woman of God.

You lived by His Word and you showed it through your actions.[10]

Many of the tributes written about and spoken of the victims have elevated Christ while declaring testimonies of love. This has transformed the role of the dead from victim to modern-day Christian martyr in the cause of Christ. This, alone, gives meaning to the perceived senseless loss and creates even more healing for our nation's injured soul. Only through God's vision can this be accomplished. We can sing "God bless America." Chinua Achebe's tragedy may never be resolved, but America's will be through the one and only "great physician." At the crossroads of the WTC crisis, God will lead the march from our helplessness to our healing. Job concludes: "But he knows the way that I take; when he has tested me, I will come forth as gold. My feet have closely followed his steps; I have kept to his way without turning aside."[11]

Chapter 15

Bittersweet Developments:
Melvin and Delvin

The phone call came in one May morning. My high school friend, pediatric ophthalmologist Dr. Irene Ludwig, was calling from the roadside in Tennessee. She had just returned from ophthalmology meetings where her colleague, also an ophthalmologist, Dr. Alan Chow, had stunned the ophthalmologic community with the invention of a silicone chip implant that brought back sight to those patients who were totally blind from retinitis pigmentosa. Irene had been keeping me posted on Dr. Chow's research for about a decade, but all along it was too early to tell whether it would be of any help to me. Though the work was elegant and sophisticated, so much had to happen before it could even be tested in humans. However, this year the trials to evaluate its safety in humans showed it not only to be safe but that it also had tremendous ability to bring back sight in some individuals. She told me that patients may only be about five years away from such an operation and even suggested that I might be aggressive about entering the experimental trials.

The news impact on the ophthalmologic world was equaled by the avalanche of emotions I felt that day, and I was more ill at ease than I had ever been about my eye condition. Why was I being so unenthusiastic in the wake of good news? I could imagine the cheers among my friends, family, and church members for such a hope, but I was racked by many questions. If I had the surgery, would it be successful? How would I adjust to being sighted after twenty years? Would my life, which has taken on so much meaning despite and possibly because of my testimony in coping with blindness, take a drastic change? Would recovering sight change my relationship with God? Would I be less dependent on Him who had been so faithful and start relying only on myself? Would I find that being sighted has its downside? How would I react when I saw myself clearly for the first time? Would I be alarmed by the aging? Would I be overstimulated by the images of things that I may not want to see?

When I arrived at my weekly Bible study, I felt as if I was delivering bad news during prayer time rather than an amazing discovery. Then it dawned on me. The one silver lining that I could safely delight in without doubt is that I would not only see my future grandchildren but also be able to take an active role in caring for them. The latter was an option that I had written off many years ago when I realized that I could no longer chase after toddlers because I did not have the vision to ensure that they were safe without another sighted person nearby. Now, if the artificial silicone implant were to work, it would change my future with respect to my family. I clung onto this thought, and it became my answer and consolation to the barrage of questions. One might think I was crazy to have such good news wreak havoc in my mental life, but the Lord knew me well. Within a week, the daily devotional guide I used spoke about an incident in which a blind man received curative surgery for his sight problem, and it was noted by his fiancée that his personal adjustment was difficult as compared to the joy of his friends and family. Thank you, God, for the reassurance that some of my ambivalence is "normal." Just help me to make the change and not be hooked on snails, as in the following fable:

A crane was wading in a stream and looking for snails to eat when a beautiful swan landed nearby. The crane had never seen a swan before, so he asked, "What are you?"

"I'm a swan," came the reply.

"And where did you come from?" the crane inquired.

"Heaven," the swan answered, and he eagerly spoke of a city of pure gold with jasper walls and pearly gates.

At that point the crane interrupted, "Tell me, are there snails in heaven?"

"No, I'm afraid not," the swan said.

"Then I don't care to go there," the crane stated decisively. "I like snails!"

Whatever happens will be a process, and just as God guided me in adjusting well to blindness, He will also guide me, if it is to happen, into sight. In order to highlight some of my insights into the process, let me share my reaction to the television program that announced the invention to the world. Melvin and Delvin were twins in their sixties who had retinitis pigmentosa and were chosen to receive the artificial implant from Dr. Chow. They were featured in a *Dateline* special program titled "Vision Quest." Dr. Chow's pioneering research with his brother, Vincent, was also being explained to the television audience. Ironically, I missed the first airing of this show because I was in Wisconsin delivering a keynote speech to a national parish nurse conference at Concordia University. It so happened that Melvin and Delvin were two hometown boys from the state of Wisconsin.

When my son woke me up several weeks later to see a 2:00 a.m. repeat airing of this show, I listened to the friendly Wisconsin banter of these two men so reminiscent of the delightful people I had met recently in that state. In spite of my blindness, I faced the television screen and listened to the interviewer describe the emotions and experiences of these twins as it led up to the surgery and what happened afterward. Because I am a blind physician and psychiatrist, I am quite used to listening for people's moods in their vocal patterns as well as in their words, and I elicited certain things from these men. Melvin, the older twin, a happily married man with five children, had heard of the research and was the first to apply for surgery. After acceptance, he then requested that his twin brother, Delvin, who also suffered from retinitis pigmentosa, receive the same opportunity. Delvin was a divorced father and businessman who had traveled and seen a great deal in his sighted life before going blind. Both spoke honestly and openly about their losses and limitations from blindness. Particularly difficult for them was the loss of independence when they were forced to give up driving. The other hardship was not being able to see the faces of their children after a certain point. Their children, now grown, all had a matter-of-fact and sometimes humorous attitude toward their respective fathers and did not seem to suffer for their parent's condition at all.

The brothers underwent the surgery. No guarantees were given for a successful outcome, and they were told that it may take a while after surgery to see any results. Furthermore, they were required not to talk to each other about the results of surgery until a month later, when they would be examined. In the end, Delvin, the younger twin, gained an incredible amount of sight, and his brother, who had first applied for the procedure, did not. This information was not revealed to the audience until near the end of the program. I knew only that it had worked in one twin but not the other. As I listened to the beginning of the *Dateline* interview, I was struck by how well adjusted Melvin seemed to be as he spoke truthfully about his anticipation of the procedure. I was equally struck by how discontent Delvin seemed at times, especially when he spoke of seeing again and his goals for the future. It was subtle, but there was a sense of tragic hesitancy in his voice.

The obvious question was: Did Delvin not regain his sight? Intuitively, I surmised that Delvin was the one who had recovered his vision, leaving his well-adjusted brother in the dark but obviously the more content of the two. I was right, and I think it was easy for me to arrive at my conclusion given my own psychological processes. I thought of the "survivor guilt" in Delvin. I picked up the ambivalence in trying to adjust to the intricacies of being sighted after decades of blindness. Even his comment—"I look *old*"—when he first saw himself in a mirror spoke volumes of the surface as well as the deeper issues that one would encounter in such a transition. The interviewer implied that Delvin's brush with death when an electrical fire burned his house down could have something to do with Delvin's upheaval, and that may very well be. However, the fire incident paints a picture of survival and points to the guilt one feels when one survives alone. Delvin has received the miracle of sight, leaving the brother who orchestrated the healing process behind. One can never take full joy and appreciation of such a wonder under these bittersweet circumstances. I thought of my own family and my younger sister, Evelyn, who also has the same eye condition. Will we be faced with these issues when the surgery becomes available? Will we be at peace with ourselves if there is a discrepant outcome? Will our love for each other, trust in God, and healthy adjustment to blindness be enough to sustain us through any discordant outcome? As Melvin and Delvin were prayerful people, I pray and hope for the best and ask for the ability to adjust to any untoward result.

As for Dr. Alan Chow, I was touched by the portrayal of his sincere dedication to finding a cure for retinitis pigmentosa motivated by the sheer frustration of watching children go blind with no hope of cure. In the two phone conversations I had with him over the years when I was in Chicago for meetings, I never saw this side of him and his brother Vincent. We merely talked about his progress with the medical science in an emotionless, scientific manner that physicians are comfortable with. In the interview, the heavy time and financial investments that he and his brother had made spoke clearly of his dedication and conviction that they would find a way. It was obvious that Dr. Chow had developed a fondness for his twin patients, even taking them out to dinner before the surgeries. It was very funny to me when Delvin, who had dreamed of seeing the face of his doctor, called Dr. Chow an "angel" when he first actually saw him. Never in my mind did I picture a Chinese angel, and being Chinese myself I would have noted any such artistic representation of angels. In my earlier sighted life I had never encountered one. But then who has ever met one to confirm the truth? I guess an angel can look Chinese.

My friend Irene's long-standing enthusiasm for the genius of Dr. Chow's work was finally confirmed.

As I deliberated these developments, I received an e-mail from the wife of missionary ophthalmologist Dr. Sam Powdrill. Sam and Rachel Powdrill serve as a medical team in Africa. It read:

Dear Elaine,

You must be seriously contemplating the new surgery to ask such questions [whether or not people have problems regaining vision]!!!

We have only seen HAPPINESS in restoration of sight. It does take time for the full impact to come to patients, and their families. We used to tell our cataract patients in England that full sight will be restored in 4-6 weeks. I always thought that was ridiculous because we knew most people were seeing 20/20 or needing reading glasses only (right) after the surgery. I realize, now, after working with this type of surgery/patient for years, that it is all the ramifications, not actually the seeing, that take 4-6 weeks. One discovers daily little things anew that you had forgotten you could see or do. I do not think you would regret it. It is frightening on this side of the surgery to think what you will look like when you haven't seen yourself for 15(?) years, but think of the joy of seeing your husband, your children, your parents, and friends, and all of God's creation again. It will be beautiful to have that sight in heaven, but God would smile to see you have it again here on earth. Maybe the surgery is not perfected yet, but your eyes are not perfect now either. Even if you gain nothing, have you lost? Your hopes would be dashed, yes, but the surgery will not make you go blind!!! We're praying for you.

Keep in touch,
Rachel[1]

I now face a new frontier in my life. As with all the other transitions I have had to go through, the Lord will be my shepherd and guide through this as well.

For "we live by faith, not by sight."[2]

Chapter 16

Unwanted Genes

Eagerly, I scanned an article from the magazine *Christianity To-day* into my computer—equipped with software for the blind—and the artificial voice uttered the contents. I heard the following poignant story:

> A morning at Silicon Valley's fast growing Grace Covenant Community Church. Members of this mostly Chinese-American congregation were aflutter about the christening of "Grace's triplets." Chinese Americans revere healthy children, and this event last year was to be a celebration. The three infants had been born to Gary and Joanne, two beloved members.
>
> But the smiles quickly faded: one of the babies had a complication. "Our son was born with Down syndrome," Joanne told the congregation in Los Altos. "We were quite deflated. There are some families that would not acknowledge this, one of the worst things [that can happen] in an Asian family."
>
> Joanne says she and her husband took their pain about their newborn son to God. Then they took their story and their burden to the church. "We feel honored God chose us to raise our son."[1]

After finishing the article, I quickly sat down to compose the following letter:

Dear Editor,

> Tony Carnes has identified an important aspect in Chinese culture with respect to the Christian pro-life movement in his

article "Embracing the Unwanted." As a Chinese-American physician who also has a handicap which might have defined me as "unwanted," I have experienced firsthand the shame that many Chinese feel regarding those that are not "physically perfect." In fact, I have experienced more discrimination from my handicap than I ever did as an Asian American raised in an immigrant family. However, God in His grace has permitted me to enjoy a rewarding professional career, raise a wonderful family, and given me a challenging ministry despite my imperfection. How glad I am that I was not aborted because of my unwanted genes![2]

Elaine Eng, M.D.
President of the Board of Directors,
Boro Pregnancy Counseling Center
Author
Alliance Graduate School of Counseling
350 N. Highland Ave.
Nyack, NY 10960

This letter to the editor sums up my fervent appreciation for God and His redemptive work in those who are imperfect, myself included. I never realized when Mr. Carnes called me in January 2002 to discuss Asians and the pro-life movement that he would ultimately write about a topic that hits such a personal nerve. By his questions over the phone, I had assumed that he wanted information about statistics and the politics or the extent of Asians interested in the pro-life movement or perhaps the roles that Asians play in legislation. To my surprise, he identified the cultural determinants of being unwanted, which raised many memories in my personal life.

I recall that, as a child growing up in New York, our rides on the subways would at times be accompanied by blind men or women who would often walk down the train with canes and Seeing Eye dogs begging for money. Some of them sang (and quite well), and others played the accordion. Leaning forward in my seat because I was fascinated by this scene, my mother would jerk me back in horror, telling me that if a blind person's cane touched me, I could go blind too. I really do not know if this is one of the numerous superstitions of her native village, but needless to say it left an impression on me until I was able to outgrow it with rational thought. Yet the notion never left me. It resurfaced in my adult life while preparing for a mission trip to the Navajo reservation: I did quite a bit of research on Navajo beliefs. Questions occupying my mind included: Will these people react to me in dismay, as my mother did to the blind beggars? Am I considered a pariah in the Navajo culture, a group not dissimilar to its Asian counterparts on the other side of the Bering Strait? I did not get the answer in my research, in mission-orientation sessions, or in the countless Tony Hillerman novels centered around a Navajo detective I read that year. Happily, however, I did get the information from Beulah, one of the Navajo women and a gifted storyteller: blind people were not considered anathema in Navajo culture. Instead, they accepted the person for who he or she was in their family. This does contrast with some of their other beliefs. For example, the Navajo people have an entrenched aversion to touching the dead or belongings of the deceased. But I did not fall in *that* category, so I enjoyed a fruitful relationship with them that summer.

The contrast between my Chinese culture's reaction and God's acceptance of me is profound. A loving God can supply all that is needed to bless the handicapped believer. He demonstrates His infinite grace in helping the disabled to function. This blindness has given me a personal testimony that seems to capture the interest of even the most distracted, harried, or hardened individual. I have shared my story literally with strangers all over the world—from the French widow who found me searching for Sainte-Chapelle in Paris, to the California student touring in Canada, to the group of African doctors at the Kenyan Christian Medical Society. There seems to be no lack of interest in what the Lord has done in my life. It so ironically contrasts with my mother's Chinese philosophy. She has removed the cane from my hands at times of public scrutiny (such as during my younger sister's wedding), and even when entering a restaurant where Chinese friends might be present. Do not get me wrong. It is not nearly as bad as the case in Tony Carnes's article, in which a Chinese couple kept their handicapped child hidden from their friends all his twenty-eight years of life.

However, the sudden disappearance of my cane, which is "my eyes," reflects at least the wish to deny my condition, if not an ambivalence about having a handicapped daughter. With God's gentle hand carving out a positive self-image in me based on how he views me, I have been able to find these memories interesting rather than hurtful. I do not take it personally because it is a cultural and psychological reaction well within the norm. Yet as an advocate of those who are handicapped and as a self-appointed teacher on this matter, I wish to articulate and present these issues. It is certain that such cultural and psychological reactions to the handicapped account for some of the discrimination and unconscious prejudices that lead to the embitterment of those afflicted. God has given me the confidence to articulate this and bring it openly to attention.

I still chuckle at the many times people have yelled in my ear assuming I cannot hear because I am blind. Whenever I am a newcomer to professional meetings, there is always this impression that I stumbled into the medical meeting by accident and need to be escorted out. Of course, there is the silence that means people are uncomfortable with my presence. This could be for many reasons—something idiosyncratic to the individual, or it may have something to do with feeling unsure as to how to communicate with me. They fear I might not be able to comprehend. What they do not know is that I comprehend well and, given an opportunity, would love to help them remove their discomfort. That is what I often do. I teach others about my limitations and what they should know if they want to work with me or even assist me. As I have told other blind people, "You are the best educators to your peers and community about your condition and how one can collaborate with you to make progress in a mutual goal." This will often work to everyone's advantage. Of course, one has to recognize that some are more teachable than others, and one needs to be quite discerning about whether to lock horns with those who are totally refractory to such an education. Some people say my behavior and matter-of-fact attitude about my limitations are gracious, but I rather think of it as displaying the grace that God has given me. I feel that He has, as Tony Carnes's article puts it, really "embraced the unwanted."

Chapter 17

The Willow in Japan

Tokyo is a bustling city, a mixture of modernity and ancient traditions. Efficiency in planning and design are observed in all aspects of life here. Space is at a premium, so the apartments, garages, packaged consumer goods, and roads and footpaths are designed to be just big enough to carry out their purpose, but to the American, the sense of space seems miniaturized. In this urban—even Western, if you will—metropolis, one cannot help but notice the time-honored oriental demeanor of the Japanese men, women, and children who march quickly with a mission. Yet they are deferential, respectful to all, especially the aged and frail. They are serenely silent even in the subways. The latter in Tokyo are amazingly immaculate, constantly being washed by scores of workers, and so timely that you can set your watch by the arrival of the trains at each station. The air in summer is forever moving with strong aquatic breezes, mixed with heat and humidity. Yet for a city, the air is not offensively polluted, again a tribute to the Japanese penchant for cleanliness. This is true for most locations, unless one walks into the fog of cigarette smoke—highlighting a habit which is excessively popular in this country. The language is lyrical, gentle, and replete with words that convey humility, gratitude, and grand acknowledgment to the one being addressed.

I stepped out of Narita International Airport with both wonder and trepidation. My daughter had been in Tokyo for exactly ten days to begin her junior year studying economics and Japanese abroad at Sophia University. She had left our home with symptoms of the typical summer stomach virus that many were having in our community. However, this malady worsened during her flight to Japan, and compounded with the jet lag, culture shock, and the airport's loss of her luggage, made for a horrendous transition. Her e-mails were increasingly worrisome and depressive. When her phone was installed, I was greeted with a torrent of uncharacteristic sobs.

> "Mom, I am so depressed that I cry every day. These spells can just hit anytime, and when I hold the tears in at school or on the subway, I can barely breathe by the time I arrive at my tiny apartment. I feel confined and lonely. There are only a few students here and I can't sleep or eat. My diarrhea is worse and I don't know what to eat. Everything is so expensive, and I feel so guilty when I try to eat in a restaurant and cannot finish my dish after a few bites. The Japanese people are not wasteful, and it is offensive to waste food, but I am too sick to take another morsel. I can't decide what to buy in the supermarket, so is it OK to eat Cocoa Crispies with milk for dinner?"

More sobs and my maternal heart was broken. Yet my psychiatrist's brain was quickly hearing the classic symptoms of a possible depression in just this one conversation: crying, insomnia, poor appetite, indecisiveness, poor concentration, and excessive guilt. When I questioned her further I discovered other signs that would total up to the nine or ten symptoms that define depression. She had excessive fatigue, pessimism or negative thinking, and anhedonia, which means loss of pleasure. The only two symptoms she did not have yet were bodily agitation or slowing and suicidal thoughts. If she had only five of these complaints for two weeks or more, she would be diagnosed with clinical depression in my office. I was *not* going to wait the two weeks for this to happen. I needed to address her physical illness, which I believed was causing all this, and to take care of her. Of course, I also had to bolster her spiritual condition, which was heroically strong as she clung onto God in her misery. She wanted desperately to find a church. She felt alone and thought she needed to talk to somebody, anybody, or everybody. Alternatively, she also felt the desire to withdraw and talk to nobody. So this sad, much skinnier, but grateful young daughter of mine hugged me as I emerged from baggage claim and entered the land of the rising sun. Would I be facing the thunderstorms of my daughter's acculturation, or would there be showers of blessings on Genevieve and me?

God is the great physician. This has been my stand in my medical career. I am just privileged to be His tool as He gives healing to the patients I treat. His healing extends from the many medicines He gives science and the many treatments or psychotherapy modalities that have value even if they are not perfect. Finally, His healing can be the result of a purely divine intervention and the answer to my fervent, consistent prayers on my patients' behalf. In talking to those who suffer, I ask God for His prescription for what to say as described in the book of Proverbs. "A word aptly spoken is like apples of gold in settings of silver."[1] Combined with good listening skills, excellent care, and patience, the work of the Holy Spirit is the foundation for therapy. I call this the biopsychosociotheological model. Can I bring this framework to my daughter and add onto it the mother's nurturance, love, and care that I really wanted to deliver?

The first two days I silenced my anxiety in order to listen so that she could have a chance to talk and ventilate all her unhappiness. I wanted her to know that I understood her suffering. She had been feeling like a failure in her adaptation because I was coming to Japan. She thought that maybe she should tough it out by herself. I reminded her that many parents accompany their children to college when they go away. My coming now did not reflect any inability on her part; I just came a week later than most parents do. She had been so independent in her freshman and sophomore years at college that we had no doubt she could manage this educational experience without us too. But we did not foresee her becoming ill at the point of departure. So in Tokyo, I cooked her favorite foods, which were now decidedly American: burgers, spaghetti and white clam sauce, and grilled salmon, because she was sickened at the thought of the Japanese foods she ordinarily craved—sushi, teriyaki, tonkatsu, etc. Her diarrhea persisted, and I reminded her that I would monitor it with her and take her to a doctor if the foods she was now eating did not help. The assurance that Mom was here to watch her gave her some peace of mind, but there was so much she had to obtain and do. In order to continue her work in school she needed an electronic language dictionary, supplies for her apartment, and a bank to exchange our traveler's checks for currency. We found that to convert these checks to yen was not as easy as we expected. It is very difficult to use any means of currency other than actual yen in Japan. Credit cards, American checks, and other monetary exchange items are not usable in many places, and she was frustrated with just trying to get money using her limited Japanese. She had encountered many rejections at stores and banks. Finally, she needed a place to worship. Where does one go in a foreign land, and can the Lord show us even in this unfamiliar place? With only prayers of pleading, heavy hearts, and my own desire to be encouraging, we asked God to show us the way to find a Christian home for Gen the next day.

That night, before she tried to go into her fitful sleep, she received an e-mail from Pastor Kim of the Shibuya Evangelical Church with an invitation and directions to go to their Sunday service. She called him on the phone and they decided that the evening service would be good for her, as English was spoken in addition to Japanese, catering to an international congregation. "By the way, Mom, he wanted to know if you would be the guest speaker tomorrow night," Gen said. "Tell him yes," I replied. This unexpected request felt powerfully like an opportunity from God for which I did not have the option to hesitate. So while Gen slept, I prepared my talk, asking God for His direction and apt words for this congregation of people, all strangers to us. Pastor Kim was a colleague of friends of mine whom I had met during their time in the United States. A French pastor and his Japanese wife, Jean-Christophe and Keiko graciously made the connection for us from their home in Paris. They were very supportive of Genevieve and knew that her adjustment in the town of Heiwadai was extremely rough. God used these dear people to find us a church at the zero hour.

Evening service, also called Shibuya Harvest Ministry, was a pleasant worship experience complete with the familiar hymns and contemporary songs that Gen and I knew well from our home church. When alternating English with the Japanese verses, I heard the lovely voice of my daughter singing in both languages, and I knew that God was continuing to strengthen and teach her how to worship Him in another tongue. Up to this point she had been too overwhelmed and anxious to use her junior high school level of Japanese that she learned in the States, but the church service gave her an opportunity to sing the words in a safe place without recrimination or ridicule. Her voice, which she had "lost" from fear and weakness, became a little stronger. After this I noticed she attempted to speak Japanese more often as the days went by. It was as if her tongue was released from the paralyzing grip of anxiety through the praiseful singing.

What does a blind woman say in one hour (with Japanese translation) to a congregation of total strangers and her sad, worried, and still somewhat sick trooper of a daughter? Is there such a message that will convey hope to her, give the listeners a clear sense of God's strength, and provide scriptural wisdom to meet the many unknown cares of this audience? The answer was decidedly YES. Pastor Kim, with his kind, sensitive conversation with Gen in his office, ended our chat with a prayer for the evening's program, and I knew I was prepared to speak a message of love with my heart, mind, and soul. My testimony—that my blindness came at just the time in my life to afford me the chance to leave my consuming OB/GYN residency and be a full-time mom—gave me the chance to tell my daughter how much I loved her and her brother. I said blindness was an answer to my prayer to be the primary nurturer and parent to them and that I considered it a gift from God. I said I would have never changed this life course even if I were given the hypothetical chance. Parenting them and being blind may seem to be bittersweet and contrasting developments, but in my case it was all for the good. The congregation heard about the moments and images I cherish in my mind's eye about those early years of my children's lives when I still had some sight left. I was hoping that Gen would hear that my love for her was a priority. She needed to know that putting all things aside to rush to her in Japan was but a small example of what a mother would gladly do, especially a mother who has seen that it is better to be blind and be with your children than to be sighted and practicing as a physician. Motherhood is a vocation—or rather a privilege—that only one person can fulfill and do wholeheartedly! The second part of my message spoke of my wall-climbing episode, which illustrates the need for perseverance in the Christian life. It can be overwhelming, frightening, and exhausting at times, but clinging to faith is the essential ingredient to obtaining the goal. Could this encouragement be useful to the church members and would it address the issues that Gen was facing? The concluding segment was devoted to the seven coping skills for anxiety found in Philippians 4:6-9.

> Do not be anxious about anything, but in everything, by prayer and petition, with thanksgiving, present your requests to God. And the peace of God, which transcends all understanding, will guard your hearts and your minds in Christ Jesus. Finally, brothers, whatever is true, whatever is noble, whatever is right, whatever is pure, whatever is lovely, whatever is admirable—if anything is excellent or praiseworthy—think about such things. Whatever you have learned or received or heard from me, or seen in me—put it in practice. And the God of peace will be with you.[2]

Slowly and steadily, I developed and repeated the seven steps in dealing with anxiety and worries that come from this passage. These seven directives also make up the basic principles of cognitive-behavioral therapy for anxiety disorders, and I have integrated them into my practice. The seven coping skills are as follows: First, stop anxious thoughts. This is counterintuitive, as most people dwell on what worries them in order to find solutions. If it is a chronic worry, such preoccupation will only make it worse by sustaining the worry loop. Instead, individuals should find techniques and practices that work for them to nip worrisome thoughts in the bud. Some people snap rubber bands on their wrists to remind themselves to get away from the anxious thought. Others visualize a big stop sign, and others just tell themselves a determined "no."

Next, they have to focus on something else, which could be another activity or, as stated in the book of Philippians, they could turn all their attention to God. The phrase "in everything" describes reshifting one's focus from worries to something else. What better focus can there be for a Christian than on the sovereign God who can provide comfort and aid?

The third coping skill is prayer and petition. This should not be limited to repetitive prayer about one's worry, as that would be analogous to dwelling on the anxious thought. Rather, the individual should resume his or her normal prayer life of adoration, intercession, confession, and thanksgiving.

The latter turns out to be the fourth coping skill. The mind can do only one thing at a time. If it is thinking about what one is thankful for, as in counting one's blessings, it will crowd out the worries. Because mood is dependent on thought in cognitive-behavioral theory, thanksgiving can bring the mood from anxiety to calm and even joy.

Fifth, the writer, St. Paul, admonishes us to think about what is true or real. Many anxious people dwell on the worst-case scenario, with "what if" thoughts making these thoughts seem real when they are statistically unlikely. Although the worried individual *knows* that his or her thinking is not realistic, he or she *feels* as if the worst is likely to happen. God tells us to believe only that which is real and set our minds on it. He listed a host of other things for a person to set his or her mind on.

One such item is to think about what is "lovely," which is the sixth coping skill called visualization. In creation, He has given each one of us lovely scenes in our memory. Visualizing them by using our imagination to bring these scenes into our mind's eye for an interval of time can be relaxing and calming.

The final coping skill is found in Philippians 4:9, and it refers to the need to "practice." We need to practice these seven skills daily, especially if we are prone to worry. One cannot give up after one try and say it does not work. The effectiveness of these skills comes only with a lifetime of practice. I reminded the audience that it will become easier with time and habitual repetition. The end result will be that God's peace will guard their hearts and minds in Christ. With this prescription for anxiety, I ended my missive of a mother's love and motivational message for perseverance. It was my hope that these words would meet the needs of the congregation as well as my daughter.

After the service, Genevieve came up to me and told me she took notes on all the seven biblical coping skills for anxiety. "Great," I said. At this point, I wanted to stay by her side and facilitate her meeting others. I was concerned that in her condition she might be too withdrawn and shy, qualities previously unknown to this child who is very adept at meeting people and making friends. I did not want to be the center of attention, but soon I was inundated by people wishing to thank me, ask questions, or discuss their problems. As much as I struggled to stay by Gen's side, I was pulled away to speak privately to someone. I was torn because I wanted to be polite and sensitive, but my priority was to ease my daughter's entry into this fellowship. When I quickly made my way back to the chapel, I was delighted to hear her conversing animatedly in English with some young people in the church. What a relief! This church was doing a lot of healing and good for Gen.

Over the earlier course of the week Gen still had many sad and anxious periods during the day. Yet the fighter in her kept going to classes and forcing herself to eat the many things I tried to prepare for her. Food shopping with the generous honorarium given to me by Pastor Kim symbolically showed her God's grace and generosity especially since we still could not find a bank to get yen from our traveler's checks and our own supply was low. When she was indecisive about buying the expensive Japanese produce, I urged her to put any food that mildly appealed to her in the cart and told her not to worry about it, as she needed proper nutrition. She needed good food to counteract her illness which left her looking like Twiggy, the British model from a previous era. Eating well now despite the expense is proper stewardship of the body God gave her, I admonished. We demonstrated hospitality to a classmate who lived in her apartment building. Gen wanted to "practice hospitality," as the Bible says, to this wonderful girl who had befriended her, and we then invited her to go shopping and spend some time with us. Besides her and the Shibuya young people, God started supplying new relationships that week—an Inter-Varsity staff member; a visiting friend from California who spends holidays with family in Japan; Yumiko, a woman who I had taught when she was studying at Alliance Theological Seminary; and other foreign students in the building who had already spent time studying at Sophia University. The ample provision of caring friends started to work to heal her withdrawn state. She started to regain her appetite and her sleep normalized. God also put us in front of a bank while we were shopping. We thought we had serendipitously found an open bank, so we walked in to inquire about exchanging traveler's checks for yen. Again they denied our request as had all the other banks we had visited, but they pointed us to one in the neighborhood that would help. It took us a while to find it, and I whispered a blind person's prayer: "Lord put our eyes on this place as we cannot tell where we are to go." Lo and behold, we were staring at a nonbanklike storefront which, to our amazement, was still open in the late afternoon. When they said they were willing to cash our $5,500 worth of traveler's checks, we broke out into a chorus of ecstasy and relief.

It turns out that the bank's name included had the surname of Yumiko's husband's corporate employer. This lovely Christian couple had helped Gen settle into her apartment the previous week. We did not find this out until we met them for dinner later in the week. However, this was Wednesday, and when we returned home, ate dinner, and got ready for bed, I sensed something was dramatically different about Gen. She had eaten all of her dinner for the first time in many days, and there was more. When she said her prayers that night, I could tell from the content that she had made the turn toward health. It was clear to me as a mother and also a psychiatrist that a significant switch had occurred. My whole body flooded with release, and the tears just flowed into my eyes as I quickly finished my own "Amen" and kissed her goodnight. I had to run to the bathroom so I could cry freely for joy so as not to worry her. As you would expect, Gen continued her recovery to health. By the time I left on Saturday, she was her usual self, the familiar confident, healthy, friendly young woman I knew. Even more, she had grown from this experience—wiser, with greater character, and with spiritual strength and the ability to weather hardship. She had a greater trust in God to help her through tough times.

Yumiko and her husband Masafumi, told us about her 101-year-old grandfather who is alive and well living with his almost-centenarian wife of seventy-six years. She told of his sagacity and his calming influence on her and the lives of many others. People enjoyed being in his company. What does it take to have such blessings of character and longevity? The grandfather says one must be like the willow tree. If one studies it, one sees how it bends with the winds and the elements with ease and strength. It is its intrinsic flexibility that gives it the power to endure and remain strongly planted. In the same way, people must acquire the suppleness to bend with the winds of life's adversities in order to remain confident and planted in the place where they should be. Just live like the willow, and you will be not only strong but also calm and unfaltering under stress. Yumiko has drawn a lot of strength from her grandfather's words. She and Masafumi themselves have gone through many transitions and hardships, and through culture shock, as they have had to live abroad in Singapore, in the United States, and now back in Japan. It is precisely the difficulties with these adjustments that made her a wonderful model and advisor to Gen in the first week. Gen had longed for Yumiko's company and conversation when she first arrived. Yumiko's grandfather teaches that if a person is climbing a mountain, he or she must have the faith to know it is done one step at a time. He or she must also believe that although the trail is long and the mountain dauntingly high, he or she must have the outlook that at some point in the future he or she will be able to look back and see that the climb is complete. We will see that we have overcome what we thought we could not do. We must be like the willow tree to have the hope of making it. Genevieve understood this teaching in a deeper way as the Tanis told us this story. She has a renewed outlook on her upcoming year in a foreign land. She e-mailed her dad back home and told him she was going to make it through the year now. As with my own life, God has transformed my daughter into the flourishing willow tree.

> Blessed is the man who does not walk in the counsel of the wicked or stand in the way of sinners or sit in the seat of mockers.
> But his delight is in the law of the LORD, and on his law he meditates day and night.
> He is like a tree planted by streams of water, which yields its fruit in season and whose leaf does not wither. Whatever he does prospers."[3]

Notes

Preface

1. *Holy Bible, King James Version* (Nashville, TN: Thomas Nelson Publishers, 1984), John 10:10(b).

Chapter 1

1. Personal communication.
2. Quotes taken from an interview.
3. Personal communication.
4. Personal communication.
5. International Bible Society, *Holy Bible: New International Version* (Grand Rapids, MI: Zondervan, 1984), Romans 8:28.
6. *Holy Bible, King James Version* (Nashville, TN: Thomas Nelson Publishers, 1984), Matthew 6:33.
7. Barbara Samaan, *"Martha, Martha": How Christians Worry:* Implications for the World Trade Center tragedy. *Journal of Religion and Health,* 2000, 41(1): 82-83.

Chapter 2

1. International Bible Society, *Holy Bible: New International Version* (Grand Rapids, MI: Zondervan, 1984), Philippians 3:13-14.
2. International Bible Society, *Holy Bible: New International Version,* Luke 10:38-42.

Chapter 3

1. International Bible Society, *Holy Bible: New International Version* (Grand Rapids, MI: Zondervan, 1984), Psalm 36:9.
2. International Bible Society, *Holy Bible: New International Version,* Romans 8:28.
3. International Bible Society, *Holy Bible: New International Version,* Psalm 4:7.

Chapter 4

1. International Bible Society, *Holy Bible: New International Version* (Grand Rapids, MI: Zondervan, 1984), Colossians 3:18.
2. International Bible Society, *Holy Bible: New International Version,* Proverbs 31:10-30.
3. International Bible Society, *Holy Bible: New International Version,* Ephesians 6:5.
4. Irvin B. Yalom, *The Theory and Practice of Group Psychotherapy,* Fourth Edition (New York: Basic Books, 1995), p. 482.

Chapter 5

1. International Bible Society, *Holy Bible: New International Version* (Grand Rapids, MI: Zondervan, 1984), 2 Corinthians 3:2-3.
2. International Bible Society, *Holy Bible: New International Version,* Hebrews 12:1-3.

Chapter 6

1. John Hughes, *Sing Joyfully* (Carol Stream, IL: Tabernacle Publishing Co., 1989), p. 442.
2. Geron Davis, *Praise Chorus Book* (Nashville, TN: Marathas Music Co., 1993), p. 148.
3. *Holy Bible, King James Version* (Nashville, TN: Thomas Nelson Publishers, 1984), 2 Corinthians 5:7.
4. International Bible Society, *Holy Bible: New International Version* (Grand Rapids, MI: Zondervan, 1984), Psalm 127:1.

Chapter 7

1. International Bible Society, *Holy Bible: New International Version* (Grand Rapids, MI: Zondervan, 1984), Titus 2:3-5.
2. Personal communication.

Chapter 8

1. *Holy Bible, King James Version* (Nashville, TN: Thomas Nelson Publishers, 1984), 2 Corinthians 4:18.
2. *Holy Bible, King James Version,* Psalm 42:1.

3. Ernie Rettino and Debbie Kerner, *Kid's Praise # 5 Psalty's Camping Adventure Album* (Nashville: Word Inc./Rettino/Kerner Pub., 1980), song, "One Step at a Time with Jesus by Our Side."

4. The Navajo Hymnal Conference, *Jesus Woodlaaji Sin* (Farmington, NM: Navajo Hymnal Conference Inc., 1979), p. 303.

Chapter 9

1. International Bible Society, *Holy Bible: New International Version* (Grand Rapids, MI: Zondervan, 1984), Isaiah 42:16.

Chapter 10

1. International Bible Society, *Holy Bible: New International Version* (Grand Rapids, MI: Zondervan, 1984), 2 Corinthians 12:9-10.

Chapter 11

1. International Bible Society, *Holy Bible: New International Version* (Grand Rapids, MI: Zondervan, 1984), Judges 6:34-40.

2. Kenyan greeting.

Chapter 12

1. International Bible Society, *Holy Bible: New International Version* (Grand Rapids, MI: Zondervan, 1984), Romans 12:15.

2. Taken from flyer for the David Stewart Lecture, February 19, 2002.

3. Personal communication from Dr. Jarrett Richardson.

4. Taken from flyer for the David Stewart Lecture, February 19, 2002.

Chapter 13

1. Personal communication from Robert Post, MD.

Chapter 14

1. International Bible Society, *Holy Bible: New International Version* (Grand Rapids, MI: Zondervan, 1984), Job 23:1-2.

2. Arline Kaplan, Psychiatrists in the Midst of Horror. *Psychiatric Times*, 2001, 17:3.

3. Chinua Achebe, *No Longer at Ease* (New York: Doubleday Books, 2000), pp. 45-46.

4. International Bible Society, *Holy Bible: New International Version,* Job 23:8-9.

5. International Bible Society, *Holy Bible: New International Version,* Job 23:6-7.

6. International Bible Society, *Holy Bible: New International Version,* Job 23:3-5.

7. Arline Kaplan, Psychiatrists in the Midst of Horror, p. 1.

8. Peggy Noonan, God Is Back. *Opinion Journal,* 2001, September 28. Available online: <http://www.opinionjournal.com/columnists/pnoonan/archive/>.

9. Sources: *The New York Times, Washington Post, Newsweek,* Associated Press, February 2001, Trial of Bin Ladin Associates Opens in New York. Available online: <http://www.ict.org.il/spotlight/det.cfm?id=560>.

10. Angela Chin, Our Loving Memories of Jennifer (New York: private publication, 2001), last page.

11. International Bible Society, *Holy Bible: New International Version,* Job 23:10-11.

Chapter 15

1. Personal communication from Rachel Powdrill.

2. International Bible Society, *Holy Bible: New International Version* (Grand Rapids, MI: Zondervan, 1984), 2 Corinthians 5:7.

Chapter 16

1. Tony Carnes, Embracing the Unwanted. *Christianity Today,* 2002, 46(May 21): 22.

2. Elaine Eng, Review of "Embracing the Unwanted" by Tony Carnes. *Christianity Today,* 2002, 46(July 8): 8.

Chapter 17

1. International Bible Society, *Holy Bible: New International Version* (Grand Rapids, MI: Zondervan, 1984), Proverbs 25:11.

2. International Bible Society, *Holy Bible: New International Version,* Philippians 4:6-9.

3. International Bible Society, *Holy Bible: New International Version,* Psalm 1:1-3.

Bibliography

Achebe, Chinua, *No Longer at Ease.* New York: Doubleday Books, 2000.

American Psychiatric Association, *Diagnostic and Statistical Manual of Mental Disorders,* Fourth Edition. Washington, DC: American Psychiatric Association, 1994.

Holy Bible, King James Version. Nashville, TN: Thomas Nelson Publishers, 1984.

Hughes, John, *Sing Joyfully.* Carol Stream, IL: Tabernacle Publishing Co., 1989.

International Bible Society, *Holy Bible, New International Version.* Grand Rapids, MI: Zondervan, 1984.

Navajo Hymnal Conference, *Jesus Woodlaaji Sin.* Farmington, NM: Navajo Hymnal Conference Inc., 1979.

Index

A CHRISTIAN APPROACH TO OVERCOMING DISABILITY

A Doctor's Story

_____in hardbound at $22.46 (regularly $29.95) (ISBN: 0-7890-2257-5)

_____in softbound at $14.96 (regularly $19.95) (ISBN: 0-7890-2258-3)

Or order online and use special offer code HEC25 in the shopping cart.